# The Way of the Peaceful Birther

## Amy Cox Jones

# The Way of the Peaceful Birther

## Amy Cox Jones

Salt of the Earth Press
Springbrook, Wisconsin, USA

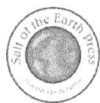

Copyright © 2010 by Amy Cox Jones. All Rights Reserved.
No part of this publication may be reproduced, stored in a retrieval system, or transmitted in any form or by any means - electronic, mechanical, photocopy, recording, or any other - except for brief quotations in printed reviews, without permission in writing from the publisher.

This book is a creative work by the author.
She is solely responsible for the content and claims therein.

ISBN: 978-0-9816949-5-5

*Editors:* Angela Eschler, Caroline Dykstra; *Design:* RiverGathering Books

Cover Photo: Jerrad Hamilton, Hamilton Photo Design.
Model: Havvah Spicer while pregnant with her daughter Haven.

Printed in the USA
2010 Printing

Salt of the Earth Press
Wisconsin, USA
www.saltpress.com

To, of course, my husband and children, with whom all this is possible and without whom my life would be empty.

AMY COX JONES has been a childbirth educator and doula since 1997. Since that time, Amy has been passionately engaged in arming couples with a more complete knowledge of their options for pregnancy, childbirth, and parenting.

# Table of Contents

**Preface** .......................................................... i

**Chapter 1** ....................................................... 1
    What Is a Peaceful Birth?
    How to Become a Peaceful Birther
    The Mind-Spirit-Body Connection
    Birthing Culture: Where We Came From and Why We're Here
    Peaceful Birthing Is Possible
    Is Natural Birth the Only Peaceful Birth?

**Chapter 2** ................................................... 29
    Limits and Possibilities
    Self-Test Pop Quiz
    Rejecting vs. Embracing the Truths that Find You
    Storytelling: Realizing What You Are Learning and Teaching
    What's Most Important: Reworking our PABC Mantra
    What Is Possible

**Chapter 3** ................................................... 68
    Taking Responsibility, Owning Your Power, Claiming Your Birthright
    Why Do You Want a Peaceful Birth?
    Raising the (Birth) Bar
    It's All Just Energy
    Just the Facts
    Ripple Effect
    Be Happy Now: Stepping Out of the PABC Mentality Today
    Extraordinary Births and Peaceful, Unexpected Outcomes

**Chapter 4** ................................................. 122
    How to Become a Peaceful Birther
    Lightbulb Moments: Personal Enlightenment and Choosing a Guide
    Why Invite a Doula
    What Do You Want Your Birth to Look Like?
    Claiming the Territory
    Of Blessingways and Babymoons

**Afterword** ................................................ 183
    Can Peaceful Births Change the World?

**Appendix** ................................................. 187
    A Brief World History of Birth—How PABC Congealed

**Footnotes** ................................................ 199

**References** .............................................. 201

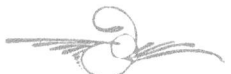

# Preface

August 2009

I have a callus on my right index finger and the joints in my right thumb are now sore and sometimes pop when I bend them, all because I had to write this book longhand—not because I think it's romantic or that I like to do things the old-fashioned way, but because I have five children that I homeschool. I also take my parenting duties very seriously, which doesn't lend itself to having blocks of time where I can sit down at my keyboard and pour out my thoughts. I wrote this book in short sections, which I consider to be an advantage because, between jotting down a sentence here or a paragraph there, I was able to think about what I wrote. I needed that time all the more because I'm writing this book primarily for my daughters and future daughter-in-law. None of them are childbearing age at present—and my daughter-in-law is yet to be identified—but I know that time will come oh so very quickly.

I have given birth five times and am in the birth field as an independent childbirth educator and birth doula since 1997, so I know that I am also writing this book for my nieces, cousins, friends, and you. Yep, that's right, I do care about you. That's the nature of hardcore birth junkies like myself. We don't care what your background is or what your circumstances are, but we do care about you, even though we've never met you, and we are passionate about spreading "the good word" of how amazing birth can be. We want everyone to experience it. Can I get a hallelujah? Amen, sistah.

I know there are ample amounts of books out there on pregnancy, childbirth, and parenting and you could be reading any one of those right now—there are many that I love and recommend—but for whatever reason you are reading this one, I thank you.

All my births have been wonderful, and each unique and special. The beauty of those births didn't happen accidentally or by chance, though. All of them were peaceful, empowering, and spiritual in their own ways. I've also attended hundreds of fantastic births, and only a few not so fantastic. I am indebted to my children, husband, midwives, colleagues, friends, family, and my clients who have allowed me into their lives to learn from them.

Now I take those lessons learned and pass them on to you. There's an admonition in our culture that says, "Each one, teach one." Truly, it's the only way that the knowledge of how to birth peacefully has been kept alive. Historically, birthing has not been written about very much; in fact, efforts to suppress its knowledge have been violent and fierce. Midwives and birthing women have a history of persecution and being imprisoned and burned at the stake. Yeah, that *might* be a deterrent to speaking up, but I'm just guessing. You've got to ask yourself, "Why has there been such an active suppression of information?" Well, that's a whole other book, I suppose, but it's certainly worth pondering.

Making this book public does involve some amount of risk. First, on a personal level, because once you proclaim to be an expert in something, you often get shown, sometimes in painful ways, just how much you don't know. Also, I am bound to get a lot of opposition. But in addition to all that, I risk ridicule and alienation from loved ones who are afraid that all I want to do is pressure them into birthing "my way." It wouldn't be too new to me, though. I've heard thirdhand—and even accidentally directly—what people, some very close to me, have said about my birth beliefs. But I don't take this to heart (anymore) because I know their adversity toward my beliefs is not a rejection of me personally. In fact, I have been lucky enough to have some of those who once kept me at arm's length later come full circle and embrace peaceful birthing.

Gratefully I learned a long time ago that by living my truth and embracing my authentic self, my greatest good will manifest. The urge to write this book only came about a month prior to my writing this now. Maybe *urge* isn't the right word. Calling? Yelling from within? Yeah, because if I consciously said, "Huh, I think I'm going to write a book," without any real urge, it would not only take forever, but it might also never get finished. It's kind of like trying to push a baby out without having the urge to push. It's an uphill battle and it's easy to give up on. I've been working on a birth project, very part time, with my neighbor for the last seven months. It's been slow going at best. Then a month ago, on a holistic mom's e-loop I've been moderating since 2002, a discussion turned misunderstanding turned argument came up.

The question that started the whole thread was, in a nutshell, "I'm 40 weeks pregnant, my doctor wants me to agree to an induction. Can I negotiate with him? What are my options?"

My response was as follows:

> Dr. XYZ is a great doctor, that is for sure, but he still has his hang ups. The last thing to go for doctors is the due date thing. Yes, there can be valid concerns and arguments for not going past 42 weeks, but they are problems that are few and far between, can be monitored and prevented, and are certainly nothing to stress a healthy mom over. Here are your options:

> 1. Go in, try to compromise (which is like trying to get a sushi chef to make Alfredo), likely not win, get the "I've seen babies become paralyzed and die" speech, get freaked out, and totally talked into an induction.
> 2. Set an induction date and show up and hope for the best
> 3. Set an induction date, pray that something comes up that prevents you from showing up (call and let the doctor know), and push the induction date forward a day or two, buying time.
> 4. Have a home birth

> You really aren't going to change Dr. XYZ's position on this. Our past clients have already tried. Not to say that there isn't a possibility, but it's slim at best. This is his philosophy combined with American Congress of Obstetrics and Gynecology (ACOG)'s position, and frankly he puts his insurance coverage in jeopardy by not doing it

*this way and risks his livelihood. I wish it were different, but unless he's willing to rock the boat, his hands are kind of tied. And again, he's one of the best OBs in town, I believe. All it takes is one bad outcome (which I know he's seen) with a mom who's at or past 42 weeks or one lawsuit, and he ain't budging. I don't mean to burst your bubble, but I think it's better just to understand your chances before going in.*

*Good luck and congrats at being so close!*

*Amy*

There was a good-sized, impassioned thread that got going from there, and it took on such a life of its own that we never did hear what she decided to do. After that exchange, as much as I tried, the thought of writing this book wouldn't leave me, even though I have everything on my plate that I do—five kids, homeschooling, a husband, classes that I teach, cooking, cleaning—you know, normal life stuff. But I put my excuses aside (after watching Wayne Dyer's *Excuses Begone!* seminar for the second time). It was something I felt I had to do. The timing was right to do it, and I trusted that I would be guided in doing so. Indeed, pockets of time have opened up for me that allowed me to get it done.

As Joe Vitale says in his book *The Attractor Factor*, "As with most things in life, there's little to be afraid of, and wealth and glory lie right around the corner. All you have to do is step forward and do the things you are being nudged to do from within." God is not just nudging me; I've been given a big push (pun intended). My children's future selves and unborn posterity are pushing me, and you are pushing me.

With humility, I hope this book becomes a best seller. I hope it becomes a classic. Not for money, fame or recognition, but because I passionately believe that every man, woman, and baby deserves a peaceful birth. It is their birthright. Your God wants you to have a peaceful birth. It's how He designed it. It's part of His plan. He wants children to be born, and the easiest way to get them here is if the families birthing them actually enjoy getting them here. What a crazy concept. It always amazes me how women who have had these horrible, traumatic births, sign up for it again without having any plans to improve upon their experience. It's a testament to the human spirit, I guess, but why not sign up for a peaceful birth the next time around?

People who have experienced empowering, peaceful births have automatically put themselves on a higher frequency than they were before. I refer to it as a shortcut to becoming a better you. My business motto is "Pregnancy, Birth, Parenting—It Doesn't Change You, It Reveals You." I've seen it happen with every birth I've attended and every baby who has come through me. The goal is to have a safe birth *and* have this whole process unveil the better parts of you. The stronger, more centered, peaceful, and powerful parts.

# 1
## What Is a Peaceful Birth?

What do you feel when you think about delivering a baby? Are you nervous? Excited? Scared? Maybe this isn't your first birth. What do you feel when you think back on your previous birth experience(s)? Did you feel safe? In control? Respected? Loved? Or the complete opposite of those emotions? Was your partner involved? Supportive? Confident? Or none of those?

Do you really believe you can achieve a peaceful birth, no matter your history or present circumstances? Regardless of what others want for you? Imagine a world where:

- All women felt empowered and loved in their birth experience.
- Both parents felt strong and connected in participating in their children's births.
- All babies were born into calm and welcoming hands.

What would that world look like?

That is the reality where peaceful birth is created and flourishes. And it is within the reach of anyone who simply begins to imagine it.

A peaceful birth can take on many different faces. It can take place in the hospital, at a birth center, in a home, or even under a tree. And despite your plans during pregnancy, if the birth strays from those plans, you can still have a peaceful birth. But the underlying commonality that births have that would classify them as peaceful experiences are that the new parents walk away from the whole of the experience empowered, happy, and content with the outcome, ready to jump into parenting with both feet.

What is the image that comes to mind when you think of what a peaceful birth looks like? Most people would say that the image puts the birthing mother as "the star" of the labor experience. She is the one being respected, attended to, and loved. No one is bullying her or talking down to her or doing things without her consent. No one is setting her needs and desires aside. When the baby is born, he is treated with gentleness and with the utmost care. The parents are the authority and caretakers of this child they have created and all present respect the power of that connection and relationship.

Most people do not understand the importance of having a peaceful birth, much less how to go about accomplishing it. But then again, most people don't believe that peaceful birthing is possible, because either they have never witnessed it, or they themselves have had a traumatic birth experience.

Most women retell their traumatic birth stories at every opportunity. These birth stories are full of drama, uncertainty, and pain. But have you ever been with someone as they retell a birth story that is free from all those elements of pain and fear? Better yet, have you ever attended such a birth? While it's great to read birth stories or watch a video of a great birth, being in the presence of someone who has experienced an empowering, loving birth is infectious. The undeniable effect that their birth has had on them is palpable. It's an especially strong energy within the first six to twelve weeks postpartum. This is one reason why I like having the couples from my previous childbirth education class series come to my current class series and tell their birth stories. It's by far one of the most effective classes in the series. No longer is it me, the authority figure, trying to engage them in learning and decision making for this esoteric event, it's their peers and it becomes more real, more tangible, more attainable. They see themselves in these new parents. And they see these new parents empowered, centered, strong, and happy.

There is a set of questions I have the new parents answer, the last of which is the most telling and impactful:

*What would you do differently next time around?*

Answers always vary, but I love it when the couple says, "Nothing. I loved how every bit of it happened." Wow. How many of your friends can say that of their births? How incredible to live your life with no regrets about this monumental experience. Don't you want that?

Even if you personally don't know someone who has done it, I want you to know that you aren't alone. Women everywhere, throughout all generations of time, have been experiencing peaceful births. There's a great-grandmother somewhere in your line who has experienced it. I guarantee that, at least. It is your birthright.

Women have been birthing on this earth for a very long time. The knowledge of how to birth peacefully has always existed, it's in our DNA and RNA. This lightbulb moment came to me when I was reading the book *The Seven Daughters of Eve* by Bryan Sykes, a professor of human genetics at the University of Oxford. In it he explains that mitochondrial DNA (MtDNA), which is genetic material inherited from your mother, has codes for the proteins necessary for energy production. MtDNA is passed unmixed from mothers to children of both sexes along the maternal line. This descent goes back to our mothers, to their mothers, until all female lineages unite. MtDNA is inherited exclusively from the mother in humans, which means that the knowledge of how to do some things, such as birth peacefully, is given to both males and females from their mother.[1]

Once this information sank in, I realized that despite our history of moving the control of birth from women to institutions and "experts," the knowledge of how to birth peacefully already exists inside of me *and* my husband. I realized that that knowledge was also lingering deep inside every person on the face of this earth. This was so empowering and helped me gain additional confidence and motivation to uncover the steps my husband and I needed to make in order to achieve our own peaceful birth. I felt like once we came across information on how to birth peacefully we would be able to recognize it, that it would resonate with us given the fact that the knowledge was already planted in us and that it would help propel us forward on our path. We just had to reconcile our internal with our external knowledge. This is a part of the reason why I know this subject matter is timeless and knows no geographic or social boundaries.

You can read story after story of amazing births, and you will in this book, but nothing can match what you experience yourself.

So, get ready to claim your birthright.

> Great things are not done by impulse, but by a series of small things brought together.
>
> ~ Vincent Van Gogh

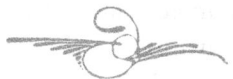

## How to Become a Peaceful Birther

I do almost all my doula consultations at my house. When I met with Jane for the first time, after we passed all the polite small talk, I asked, "So, what kind of birth do you want?" To my surprise, I caught her off guard. I think that she expected me to tell her what kind of birth she should have.

"I don't know. I mean, a good one, I guess."

"Okay. What does 'good' mean to you? What does that look like?"

"I'm not sure," Jane said, a little embarrassed.

"Well," I said, "let me ask you a question. There are endless ways your pregnancy, birth and postpartum could go. Why do you think you haven't thought about how you want it to unfold?"

"Huh. It looks like I have some work to do," Jane admitted.

I commended her for taking the first step—wanting a good birth, even though she didn't really know what that meant. She came to me at the recommendation of a friend who had said that I would help her have a good birth. And I wanted to help her, but I wasn't going to plan it for her. That actually ensures her a very *un*satisfying birth. Planning the birth for her would have taken her power from her and would have only led to a feeling of detachment.

Truth be told, Jane had a fundamental problem that if she didn't resolve now would lead not only to disappointment in birth, but also to a lifetime of disappointing experiences. She had a fear of taking responsibility and doubted her own abilities. This showed up in the form of trying to hand over her birth to someone else. Whether it was an obstetrician, anesthesiologist, midwife, doula or a bump on a log, it didn't matter. She wasn't going to have a peaceful birth, let alone a happy one, until she took responsibility for herself, her baby and her choices, committed 200 percent to them, and decided that she could do what she set out to do.

If you don't decide what you want and go for it, someone else will be eager to decide for you, and you will not become the strong, empowered woman that you can be. Allowing others to usurp your agency and make decisions for you is the antithesis of peaceful birthing. Taking responsibility and gaining confidence in your abilities is the most important, most vital step on your journey, because it is the first one. It is the foundation of a peaceful birth. Without it, no matter how the birth turned out, you will not be fully happy.

Commitment is the second step in achieving this goal. I remember once, during a childbirth education class I was teaching, when I was going over the risks and benefits of the most common birth interventions. One exchange I overheard between a couple has always stuck with me.

I had wrapped up going over all the pain medications that might be offered and I overheard one husband ask his wife, who had already had two typical, medicated births, "What do you think? Do you want to do it natural?"

"Well, I can try," she said.

At that moment, it was as if someone had jumped inside my body and taken control of my thoughts and mouth, "When you guys got engaged, did you tell him that you'd *try* to stay married to him?"

Everyone started laughing, but I was totally serious.

"Having a natural childbirth is kind of like staying married. If you told him that you'd only try to stay married, do you think he would have married you?"

"No way," the husband interjected.

His wife explained, "Well, I wouldn't even expect him to marry me. In fact, I wouldn't have even gotten married, I know myself too well. I wouldn't have stayed married if I had gone into marriage with that attitude."

"Exactly," I said, "I'll *try* to have a natural birth? No, you won't."

Luckily, this couple took my unfiltered comments well, and she actually went on to have a great unmedicated birth and subsequent fourth peaceful birth. Of course, a commitment to a certain way of birthing is no guarantee it will come to fruition, but without that commitment your chances are slim to none that it will happen.

When you are definite about having a peaceful birth and how to go about doing that, you are on your way to achieving it.

*Do or do not, there is no try.*
—*Yoda*

## The Mind-Spirit-Body Connection

*Garbage in, garbage out.*
*You get what you give.*
*That's bad/good karma.*
*Obey the Golden Rule.*

These are social mantras that most of us are familiar with. What do these mantras have to do with birth? How *do* you manifest a peaceful birth? Luckily, there has been a lot of research which has given us tools to understand just how to accomplish that. But just because science and research is "proving" these facts now doesn't mean that we haven't always had the tools to create peaceful births.

We've all heard of the placebo effect. And for the most part, people just accept that the placebo effect is real and it happens, no questions asked. What floors me is, why are there no questions asked? Here's a statement you may have heard on the news: "A new study was done that showed X drug worked 50 percent of the time, and the other 50 percent was cured by placebo."

And the reporter moves on, as if what he just said about placebo has no relevance. Just glosses right over it, as if something amazing didn't happen within that study. Having any condition improved by a placebo effect I think is amazing. Why aren't these placebo effects being treated as amazing? Why aren't we looking into and applying the placebo effect everywhere?

A placebo is basically a pill or treatment given to someone, and the pill is either a sugar pill or the treatment never happened at all. The placebo effect is when a person, thinking they have received the actual pill or treatment, recovers as if they had gotten the actual treatment.

Act as if, and it will be. Because the mind is convinced completely that something will heal the body, the body then heals. In a nutshell, that's what the placebo effect is. Everyone knows it happens. Doctors and scientists know it happens. We all know it's real, yet no one seems to take it seriously because mainstream science and culture doesn't know what to do with it. Mainstream science is just now beginning to take the mechanics of the placebo effect seriously and they are seeking to understand it. But because mainstream science and culture don't validate it, does that make it any less real or applicable? Of course not.

For example, as early as 2002, through the Freedom of Information act, there were researchers looking into the issue of the placebo effect and antidepressants. One *USA Today* article said:

> *More than half of the 47 studies found that patients on antidepressants improved no more than those on placebos. . . . [University of Connecticut psychologist Irving Kirsch said,] "They should have told the American public about this. The drugs have been touted as much more effective than they are."*[2]

Think about that. Half of the studies said that a fake pill worked just as well as the real one, with no side effects and no cost.

Another study was conducted on 40 Parkinson's patients. All agreed to and were prepped for surgery and wheeled into an operating room. All were cut open and stitched up, but only half received the neuron transplants that the surgery was being performed for. Twelve months post-surgery, those who thought they received the transplant reported better quality of life than those who thought they received the sham surgery, regardless of which surgery they actually received. In fact, one of the patients that had received the sham surgery said that before the surgery she had not been physically active for years. Afterward she resumed hiking and ice skating, believing that she had received the transplant.[3]

I also remember one birth I attended where the woman had been laboring hard at 6 cm for quite a while and was exhausted. At one point she kept on stating how all she wanted to do was sleep. I had this wacky idea to just tell her she could, "After this next contraction, go ahead and sleep, we won't wake you up until it's absolutely necessary." She fell sound asleep, even snored! When she woke up 3 minutes later, she asked how long she slept. I told her 10 minutes, "Wow, that felt great! Can I do that again?" I assured her that she could and she should sleep even longer. We repeated that about six times until she felt well rested. In her head she had slept for an hour, even though it was only a total of 18 minutes or less. She felt completely refreshed by it.

This information is so powerful! So, what is this powerful medicine, the placebo effect? It is your beliefs manifesting into real, measurable effects. Your thoughts do make up your reality.

So how does the energy of thought and belief translate into creating your physical reality? We've all heard Einstein's equation $E=MC^2$, but I don't think the majority of us are aware of its implications and meaning, because if we did, birth and our world would be operating much differently. Before the $E=MC^2$ discovery, science operated on the Newtonian theories that the universe was made up of solid objects (atoms) that were the building blocks of nature and were attracted to each other by gravity. To a large extent, this is still what is taught in school today.

What $E=MC^2$ proved, though, is that atoms are made up of smaller particles (subatomic particles), and all subatomic particles are made up of energy, nothing solid at all, even though they looked solid. So, $E=MC^2$ states that all things broken down in their most basic form is all the same thing: energy.

So, everything that is in existence—the moon, the grass, your house, colors, sound, food, medicine, yourself—is all made from the same vibrating frequency of energy that merges with other energies of the same frequency to shape our perceived reality and physical experiences.

Another scientist, Niels Bohr, believed the energy was made up of both subatomic particles and waves that had the potential to take on various forms, and this paved the way for what we know now. He believed particles appeared to be solid because of the high rate of frequency they were vibrating at.

Since the very early 1900s, the study and science of quantum physics—with Bohr being one of the influential contributors of it—has given us invaluable insight into how our thoughts shape our reality. Simply put, quantum physics (also referred to as quantum mechanics and quantum field theory) is the study of the behavior of matter and energy, and it demystifies the process of manifestation. It explains how everything comes into existence, searching for the spring from where they come from.

To apply it to our lives, you will probably have to consider setting aside what we, as a society, have been conditioned to believe about cause and effect and how our reality comes about. Quantum physics says that everything in the universe is made of the same thing: energy. And that energy basically knows no boundaries. There are some particles in the universe that do not obey the laws of physics. Bohr noted one incredible thing: this rebellious energy he was doing experiments on was always affected by the experimenter's thoughts. Even in double-blind experiments this proved to be true. His experiments revealed that if the scientist was expecting the energy to appear in the form of a wave, it would be a wave, but if he was looking for it to take on the form of something else, a "particle" (matter) is formed. The thoughts and perceptions of the scientist doing the observing determined which one it was, waves or particles.[4]

As modern-day epigenetisist and biologist Bruce Lipton puts it, subatomic particles and cells are like microchips that download the messages we give them—thought, matter, light, hormones, etc.—much like a computer program, and then take on various forms according to the beliefs we adopt.[5]

I know, "whoa" is right. When you grasp this knowledge, it can fundamentally change your life. Yes, your thoughts, emotions, and beliefs have a real, measurable outcome. This is empowering knowledge! Because now you know that *you* are the most important variable in improving the quality and outcome of your pregnancy, birth, parenting, and life!

Additionally, almost all religions place emphasis on positive thoughts as a means to attaining temporal progress. For example:

In Christianity: *As a man thinketh, so is he.*

In Buddhism: *All that we are is the result of what we have thought.*

In Hinduism: *Whatever is sown must be reaped sometime and somewhere. This is the law: every action, every intention to act, every attitude bears its own fruit. A man becomes good by good deeds and bad by bad deeds.*

From the Kabbalah: *Three are the dwellings of the sons and daughters of Man. Thought, feeling and body. When the three become one, you will say to this mountain "move" and the mountain will move.*

So, what this all means is that what the most influential religious and spiritual teachers and scriptures have been trying to teach us for thousands of years is true; we are all one, we are all made up of the same energy.

This means that your thoughts create your reality. Your thoughts, the initial energy wave forms, transform into subatomic particles that take shape based on your thoughts, emotions and beliefs, and that the energy from your thoughts and beliefs join and manifest in our physical reality, which leads us to the law of attraction

The law of attraction is the law by which thought correlates with its object. It ensures that whatever energy (anything from physical energy to thought energy) that is broadcast out into the universe is attracted to energies that are of an equal or harmonious frequency, resonance, or vibration (energy).

All of your thought waves turned particles seek other particles that match its frequency, or vibration, and in turn all these particles collide and make up physical things that we can touch and feel.

There have been experiments where DNA is extracted from someone, and as that person changed emotions, the DNA that was outside his body responded to and mirrored the emotional shifts that were happening within him, even when the DNA was hundreds of miles away. Space (how far the DNA was from the subject) and time (there was no delay) had no claim on the reaction of the DNA to its source.[6]

This knowledge, combined with your spiritual/religious beliefs, if any, becomes pivotal in grasping the importance of the visualization techniques I put forth in future chapters, and also staying in the place of love and peace, etc, that I talk about.

Many times in the book, I also refer to surrendering. We've all been in a situation where we feel like we're being "pecked to death," so to speak. Whether it's from an impatient child or nagging spouse or friend, we all know that when someone demands and forces an issue with you, you become increasingly less willing to do whatever it is that person is asking you to do as the "pecking" goes on and intensifies. That nagging is a sign of distrust and actually repels what we want. But when those around us are patient and trusting of us, we are more likely to want to meet their requests, and in most cases we go above and beyond what they ask of us.

Asking for and seeking after what you want and then fully surrendering and accepting whatever shows up in your life will actually increase the rate at which good comes to you. Then if you learn that all things can work together for your good, you will experience a greater sense of calm and peace. Also, by redefining "good" and "bad," it liberates us from our narrow belief system and helps attract peace to us. What some would consider "bad," such as cancer or death or poverty, others might not define as bad at all, but merely a steppingstone or doorway to realizing their full potential. It's very common to hear things such as, "Losing my house was the best thing that ever happened to me," or "If it weren't for my illness I would have never found my true passion in life." Within every problem there is a solution. Within every failure there is a success. Within every heartache there's a joy. When you look for the good in bad situations, you are aligning your frequencies with the good and will find solutions and joy more quickly. Through surrendering, you will soon discover that you are more likely to experience what you desire.

There are also a few times when I will refer to God. You may use whatever you feel comfortable with in place of the word God; Higher Power, Source, the Universe; whatever that may be.

> The oak sleeps in the acorn; the bird waits in the egg. . . . Dreams are the seedlings of realities.
> —James Allen
> As a Man Thinketh

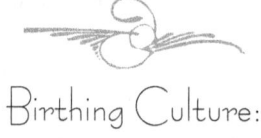

# Birthing Culture:
# Where We Came From and Why We're Here

The sources for this chapter can all be found in the timeline in the Appendix.

There has always been an interest in controlling birth. Long before we handed it over to hospitals and doctors, there was religion and government worming their way into every facet of birth as best they could. Most women and midwives did their best to protect the life and psyche of the birthing woman and baby, but when it comes to matters of life and death, history has shown us that those in authority are always trying to control them.

Up until AD 500, birth was pretty much left in the hands of the women and midwives. From AD 500 until about AD 1500, during the middle ages in Europe, male barber-surgeons began trying to monopolize childbirth services. Women were forbidden to practice medicine or midwifery and many midwives were accused of being witches and killed. Soon the barber-surgeon was delivering most, but not all of the babies.

Beginning in the 1600s bishops in the Church of England were the first to legislate control over midwifery. They were concerned with preventing witchcraft and abortions, and they also wanted to ensure that midwives were loyal to decrees of the church and state regarding birth. Civil licensing and attitudes toward birth in the American Colonies mirrored what was happening in Europe. The predominant belief stemming from the church was that labor pain was woman's punishment for Eve's sins.

In the 1700s men attending births started looking for clinical teaching material and offered their services for free to poor women. At the same time upper-class families began to rely on male doctors as primary caregivers. Men started medical schools and exclusively degreed other men in midwifery, thereby creating a male midwifery boom starting in the mid 1750s. Men became doctors merely by attending births and being quizzed later. As a result of their lack of training, childbed fever, which was caused by the doctor not washing his hands between exams or operations, killed approximately 20 percent of birthing women.

It wasn't until about 1860 when the medical community stopped blaming unwed mothers and overcrowding for childbed fever deaths and finally listened to chemist Louis Pasteur and admitted that their lack of sanitation was to blame—this after years of his being an outcast. It was also in the mid-1850s that the use of ether anesthetic during birth became fashionable both in England and its colonies as a result of Queen Victoria singing its praises after using it for the birth of her seventh child.

Changes came on rapidly starting around 1900. The first clinic Cesarean section was performed in Boston, and scopolamine and twilight sleep anesthesia, as well as forceps and episiotomies, soon became routinely used by doctors whether the woman was birthing at home or the hospital. As a result, birth injuries and deaths increased. Also notable was that the medical profession had won stronger licensing laws, and subsequently the United States Government started to become involved in maternity health care. Only about 5 percent of women, the most wealthy sector, were birthing in hospitals, but the government tried feverishly to control the many immigrant midwives who were practicing illegally in America in the early 1900s.

During the 1920s obstetrician Joseph DeLee, who was the author of the only obstetric manual at the time, set the tone for American obstetrics as we know it today. In effect, he polluted the attitude of the medical profession, and societal attitudes followed suit, with the belief that the act of childbirth was a ticking time bomb ready to explode at any second. Childbirth, in DeLee's view, was inherently abnormal and the mother was a broken vessel and a danger to her unborn child and therefore fully reliant on the obstetrician and technology to save her and the baby from this most treacherous of human conditions. As we moved into the 1930s and the American College of Obstetrics and Gynecology (ACOG) was formed, nurse midwives (mostly black granny midwives in the rural South), were tolerated because obstetricians were both unwilling to attend poor and indigent women and unable to reach rural and isolated women.

In the mid-1950s, in response to the U.S.'s high maternal and infant mortality and morbidity rate and cruel treatment of women and babies in hospitals—such as using maternal ankle and wrist restraints and performing surgery on infants without anesthesia—a very small number of humane birth and infant advocates began to appear. These included La Leche League, Dr. Grantley Dick-Read, who wrote *Childbirth without Fear;* Dr. Fernand Lamaze; and Dr. Robert Bradley, founder of the Bradley Method. As we moved through the 1960s and '70s and the mortality rates began to stabilize due to greater access to improved sanitation, availability of antibiotics, and safer Cesarean and other birth practices, the U.S. saw an almost complete shift of the care of birthing women and newborns into hospital institutions and to doctors. During this same time, however, there was a small grassroots movement from the hippie counterculture to claim their births on their own terms, primarily at home and unmedicated, which created the demand for the first birth center in 1975 and the establishment of a few lay midwives serving the middle class across the country. Surprisingly, it wasn't until 1979 when the first studies on anesthesia in childbirth were being conducted.

The 1980s and 1990s saw many changes in the birth climate. Government and insurers became heavily enmeshed in establishing who should be allowed to legally attend birthing women, how those providers should practice, and how they should get paid and from whom. During this time, though, the infant and maternal mortality rates rose. The use of induction and Cesarean increased while the use of forceps and episiotomies decreased. Alternative birthing practices, such as waterbirth, natural birth, doulas, midwives, and home birth rose as ACOG put more and more restrictions on hospitals, doctors, and birthing women. All in all, there was an effective tug-of-war going on between what women were demanding and what the American birthing establishment was willing to give them.

This leads us to where we are today. The U.S. has inherited many of the issues from the 1990s, and our Cesarean and mortality rates are obscene in comparison to other first-world countries. Women are demanding more disclosure and information from their caregivers and birthplace, as well as more compassionate and more individualized care. As alternative birthing practices continue to increase in the 2000s, ACOG (who in 2009 changed their name from the American *College* of Obstetrics and Gynecology to the American *Congress* of Obstetrics and Gynecology) is finally beginning to backpedal on decades' long protocols, such as their policies on electronic fetal monitoring, continuous IV drips in labor, and eating and drinking in labor. As many see this as an encouraging step forward in handing the power of birth back to women and increasing safety, others see it as too little too late and wonder how many more women and babies will suffer at the hands of caregivers implementing the unstudied, unscientific, and outdated medical practices to which they still hold true.

A term I use a lot to describe where we are now is "Predominant American Birth Culture" or PABC. Today's PABC is one full of fear, drama, doubt, impatience, sickness, hardship, criticism, insecurity, unnecessary pain, and risk; but it also tries to promote the fact that the birth experience has some joy surrounding it, namely the baby that results.

Those who choose to move out of the PABC and into peaceful birthing increase their odds of experiencing:

1. Miracles. I've seen countless of them. The miracles I've witnessed only happened in the births where the parents-to-be have been peaceful birthers.
2. Increased ease and comfort. The PABC of fear, sickness, doubt, etc., by the very nature of those behaviors and mindsets, produce more emotional and physical pain in childbirth than necessary and is responsible for a national Cesarean rate of 32 percent[7]. These emotions literally prevent you from moving into your right brain enough to release adequate amounts of the hormones you need to birth your baby in a peaceful way—vaginally, at least.
3. Safer delivery. First of all, refer to number 2.; also, since the '70s, a number of doula studies[8] scientifically support the fact that a peaceful birth equals a safer birth.
4. Stronger relationship with baby and spouse. When you, your partner, and baby are able to release the hormones designed to be produced and released during birth—namely oxytocin, pheromones and prolactin—you literally exchange these hormones and bond more deeply. It engenders the love, bond, and strength needed to weather difficult times together.
5. Better self image. I've never known a woman to walk away from a peaceful birth saying, "I feel horrible about

myself." "I feel broken." "I am weak." When you birth peacefully, you feel like a warrior, you feel like you're on top of the world. You feel transcended—and I'm not exaggerating. The veil between heaven and earth thins, and you catch a glimpse of pure joy and peace. No drug can produce a better high.

6. A strong legacy. Everyone leaves their stories behind, either to their posterity or the world. What is your birth legacy going to be? Just last night I was sitting around with sisters, nieces, my aunt, and my mother talking birth stories, mostly my deceased grandmother's. Some were empowering and happy, others were tragic and depressing. Your births are something you and your children will be talking about long after you have left this earth. What do you want to give them? What do you want them to take away from your stories? Strength? Weakness? Inspiration? Fear? What is your birth legacy going to be? If you say, "I don't care," think again. You will care, and it will make a difference to your posterity.

7. Parenting confidence. Imagine starting off a marriage in emotional pain, confusion, fear, sadness, and doubt in yourself. Sounds like a recipe for failure, eh? Can it be overcome? Sure. Is there an increased chance your marriage might be fraught with hardship? Yep. Starting off your parenting experience in the same way leads to an overall risk of detachment (handing your baby over to others to raise, figuratively and literally speaking), resentment, regret, and lack of confidence in your intuition. You deserve more. Your baby deserves more.

8. Respect of self and of others. The last time I heard a woman's partner say of this new mother after a peaceful birth, "Ah, that wasn't a big deal, I could totally do that." was, um . . . never. People, in particular men, stand in awe of women when they witness birth, especially a peaceful birth. It takes work, courage, and a connection with God. It's a huge deal, and men are overcome with gratitude and respect when they are involved in this process. Women also respect themselves. Peaceful birthers often respond strongly to PABC negativity with,

"I'm sorry, what are you telling me I can't do?! Have *you* ever birthed a 10-pound baby into your partner's hands after 18 hours of labor and multiple birth positions? No? Okay, then get out of my way."

When I was pregnant with my first and I casually mentioned to one of my friends what my plans were for the birth, she stifled a laugh and then tried to compassionately tell me not to get my hopes up. After all, she had birthed five babies, and she knew what this was all about. She had had everything from a natural birth to a vaginal birth after Cesarean (VBAC) and a lot in between. She warned me with the best of intentions; she didn't want me to feel like a failure when I changed my plans mid-labor. Well, not only did I stick with my plans, but I had a fantastic time because I put in a lot of work and time to make it so. Let's just say, there were no stifled laughs from my friend after that.

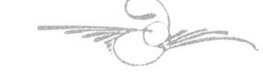

## Peaceful Birthing Is Possible

*A Grandfather from the Cherokee Nation was talking with his grandson.*

"A fight is going on inside me," he said to the boy. "It is a terrible fight between two wolves."

*The young grandson listened intently.*

"One wolf is evil, unhappy, and ugly: He is anger, envy, war, greed, selfishness, sorrow, regret, guilt, resentment, inferiority/superiority, false pride, coarseness, and arrogance. He spreads lies, deceit, fear, hatred, blame, scarcity, poverty, and divisiveness.

"The other wolf is beautiful and good: He is friendly, joyful, loving, worthy, serene, humble, kind, benevolent, just, fair, empathetic, generous, honest, compassionate, grateful, brave, and inspiring resting wholeheartedly in deep vision beyond ordinary wisdom."

*Grandfather continued;* "This same fight is going on inside you, and inside all human beings as well."

> *The grandson paused in deep reflection and recognition of what his grandfather had just said. Then he finally cried out deeply, "Grandfather, which wolf will win this horrific war?"*
>
> *The elder Cherokee replied, "The wolf that you feed."*[9]

As I mentioned before, the vast majority of births I've attended, in addition to my own, have been peaceful births. And yet I've had labor and delivery nurses say to me, "You're just lucky. If you saw what I saw, your opinion might be different. Not all births can be these pie-in-the-sky rosy experiences. Get real."

Would my opinion truly be different if I saw what they saw? I'm a firm believer that your outer reality is a reflection of your inner self.

Presently our PABC system, namely hospitals (although it certainly isn't exclusive to hospitals), just aren't set up to create a peaceful birth. Of course there are exceptions to this. Certain areas of the country are proof of that, and I've attended very peaceful births within the confines of the PABC. I myself have birthed peacefully within the PABC system! But no one who is entrenched in, dependent on, and committed to the survival of the PABC system would say that it is set up to meet the needs of a peaceful birther. The mission of the PABC is a live mother and baby, and their path to a live mother and baby does not care if the birth experience is peaceful or drama-filled. Every organization has a hidden mission, as my husband would say. The hidden mission of every organization is survival, and doing whatever they need to do to ensure that survival. In some centers, you are considered a risk taker and renegade for protecting the needs of a peaceful birther. The PABC is set up for efficiency, for profit, for the convenience and needs of the staff. It's the only way they think they can survive. It's not like they want to put your needs and desires second, third, fourth, or indeed last, but it is what it is, at least for today and since about the year 1900. They consider it a necessary evil, and most working within these places wish it could be different. But if you want a live baby at the end of it all, it's just the way things are. It's the nature of birth, they say; it's inherently dangerous, you are told.

Improving the PABC takes a movement outside of itself. If you take into account the short history presented and how we got to this point, I hope it is clear to you that it takes a grassroots movement to change the PABC into one of faith, trust, and peace with the pregnancy, birthing, and parenting process. I've observed that it takes years to implement permanent change within the PABC. For example, once it was announced by ACOG that routine episiotomies were dangerous, it took many years before it became the norm to not do them. In fact, I've witnessed some OBs who are still to this day unwilling to abandon doing routine episiotomies in their practice, something ACOG encouraged OBs to abandon back in 1983[10]. So, while it's great that things improve and change over time, you are not afforded the luxury of time. You have to go forward, and find a caregiver who supports those birth practices that resonate with you. You do not have time for practices and science to catch up with what you feel is right for you.

In no way am I trying to vilify ACOG, hospitals or their birth centers, labor and delivery nurses, or hospital based caregivers like OBs. They in fact are trying desperately to create the best birth they know how within a broken system and given the limited knowledge they posses. The problem is that they aren't taught, shown, or given the research and tools that show that the safest births are also the most peaceful, autonomous, nature-harmonized births. They have been taught that to have a safe outcome they need to value intervention, conquer and overcome nature, and control the uncontrollable namely out of fear—fear of death, fear of liability, fear of loss of income. Thanks to our cultural birth history, primarily influenced by Joseph DeLee's attitudes, bias, and beliefs, they have been taught and believe that the safest way to come out of the birth process with a live mother and baby is for you to essentially hand over your decision-making power and body to achieve it.

That's not to say that there isn't the rogue nurse who's birthed outside the hospital, or the renegade doctor who is quietly bucking the system. They are there. Most of the doulas in your area know who they are.

Over my years of doula-ing, the hospitals in the valley I lived in took turns being our favorite hospitals, all because of the nurses. Where there were two or more nurses that we knew held birthing integrity as a priority, we would encourage our clients seeking a peaceful hospital birth to go there. We kept in close contact with each of the other doulas in town, gave feedback on the staff, and would communicate where and which nurses were most favorable, so we knew going in who was likely to go to bat for us.

These nurses, and to some extent even the more open-minded doctors and certified nurse midwives (CNMs), are very careful about being too vocal, though. It's risky to speak up and defend a birthing mother's desires too much socially and in terms of keeping their job. You see, the PABC, and maybe even your social circles, suffer from something called the Tall Poppy Syndrome. The Tall Poppy Syndrome originates from accounts in Aristotle's *Politics* and Livy's *History of Rome* and is commonly referred to in Australian and New Zealand politics and media. The modern-day definition of this syndrome is that others try to denigrate any person who stands out from the crowd by being successful. It stems from Colonial days when prisoners were sent to Australia, but really the Tall Poppy Syndrome can be seen in many other cultures, and even has other terms assigned to it.

For instance, in Scandinavia there's a concept called *Janteloven*. Some of the rules of Janteloven are, "Don't think you know more than we do." "Don't think you are better than us."

In Japan, there's *Deru Kui Wa Utareru* which can be roughly translated as "the nail sticking up gets hammered down."

Crab Mentality, or Crab in a Bucket Syndrome, which stems from India, describes how when crabs are in a bucket together they grab at each other in a useless "king of the hill" competition, which ensures none escapes and there is a collective demise instead.

Sound familiar? It's a sad phenomenon that keeps people oppressed and in fear. And in fact, I find most people do this to themselves. Each of us may at one time think to ourselves, "Don't speak up, don't stand out from the crowd, don't try something new."

Conversely, take into account the International Peace Study. This study was conducted during the war between Israel and Lebanon in the early 1980s. Groups of trained people were placed amidst bombing and fighting. These groups of people mediated on the feelings of peace and love. What happened was that the fighting, the bombing, the crimes, and hospital admissions reduced exponentially in the war-torn regions. All kinds of controls were in place so that they were sure they weren't coinciding with anything like holy days or lunar cycles. What prompted this experiment were previous studies conducted in the same manner in cities across the U.S. The result was the same as for the experiment conducted during the war. The experiments were conducted repeatedly to ensure that the results were valid. They found that the threshold number of people needed in order for the experiments to work was the square root of 1 percent of the given population. So, for example, in a population of 1 million, the number of people required to effect this kind of change is only 100.[11] What a small group to effect such change! Some people also refer to this as the hundredth monkey principle.

My nurse friends' remarks to me of "Well if you saw what I see, you wouldn't be so naive" may hold a lot of weight for them personally, but what I wish is that they would choose to see what others outside the PABC see. The fact is, if they shifted their environment, paradigm, and mindset, *they* would be the ones changing their opinion. Deep down, I think they know that, because I've never met or known anyone to go from a deep-seated conviction to peaceful birth switch over to adopting the beliefs of the PABC, the reverse is almost always true. It's not that some have more willpower than others, that some are smarter than others, that some are just luckier than others, or have a higher pain tolerance than others; it's that some are ready for progress and others are not.

Some may argue that because I haven't seen every tragedy possible in birth firsthand, that somehow I am naive and unqualified to speak from a place of authority. If that were the case, than no OB or midwife would be an authority or trustworthy until they have handled every tragedy possible. While it's true you want some level of experience met, there is no way one can possible prepare themselves for every eventuality that may come their way. One of my midwives, Kaye Bullock (midwife for 25 years and thousands of births), once said something to me that has always resonated with me:

> When you know what is within the range of normal like the back of your hand, you will recognize the slightest bit of abnormality before it actually becomes a problem.

The truth is, I have seen many abnormal things begin to happen in labor and birth, and for 98 percent of those situations we used time-tested techniques and pure love to turn those situations around before they became a problem. And for those situations that weren't able to be turned around, I've still handled them beautifully and without adopting the belief system of PABC—that every woman is a potential surgical patient and/or lawsuit.

These births that had unexpected outcomes, they've been so unique and rare that no one could have prepared for the bulk of what happened anyway. Prepared or not, staying in faith and peace has always facilitated the best possible outcome for that situation.

Whenever you feel like an authority figure is trying to usurp your power and "cut the tall poppy," remember that you don't need to know everything in advance in order to make the right decision in the moment. While I do advocate for you to get all the learning you can to prepare for your birth, in truth you cannot possibly prepare yourself for all the possibilities. If you can stay in a place of peace, even amidst a crisis, your inner voice will always tell you what to do. Fear (doubt) and faith (peace) come from two polar opposing sources. Faith will always guide you to your highest good and can be accessed through listening to your gut. Every birth is different, and the outcome is never guaranteed, but every birth can be peaceful if we choose. We all have a path and lessons to learn from God in birth and you can learn them if you don't suppress, distract, or numb yourself out of it. You are meant to be that tall poppy; don't let anyone cut you down.

> For God hath not given us the spirit of fear, but of power, and of love, and of a sound mind.
> —2 Timothy 1:7

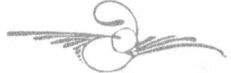

## Tuba City: Is This Hospital in America?

Tuba City Regional Hospital in Arizona is doing it. Doing what, you ask? They are creating a PABC worthy of many praises in their community.

The hospital is run by the Navajo Nation, and even though it could stand to use some updating and funds, they are outperforming most hospitals, especially "rich" hospitals, hand over fist.

What sets Tuba City apart are a few things. Primarly staffed by C.N.M.'s who are there around the clock and hands on, they tout a cesarean rate of only 13.5%. Considering the national cesarean rate is 32.3%, I'd say they are doing something right! Not only that, but their VBAC rate is 32% - far better than the national average.

One other aspect which I think is really the defining factor in setting this hospital apart form the rest of the country, is their culture. Because the hospital is run by, and primarily serves, a community of people who collectively view childbirth as a primarily spiritual and family centered experience, emphasis is placed on those very real aspects of love and peace, which translates into healthy outcomes.

Navajos generally want more than two children, so they want to avoid anything that might reduce those odds, namely unnecessary cesareans. Additionally, they see any type of cutting an invasion to the spirit. Families, including children, are invited into the birth experience, so birth is a very normal, welcomed event in the Navajo culture. Women in the community know how to care for the woman in labor and take on that role of doula willingly.

This country can learn much from this humble, dusty hospital in Arizona. Peaceful birthing in the hospital can become a PABC if we collectively value it.[12]

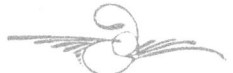

# Is Natural Birth the Only Way to Peaceful Birth?

Women have learned collectively, though not necessarily consciously, to fear the birth experience, and every obstacle has been put in our collective paths to keep us from experiencing its majestic power.

Imagine what might happen if the majority of women emerged from their labor beds with a renewed sense of power of their bodies, and of their capacity for ecstasy through giving birth. When enough women realize that birth is a time of great opportunity to get in touch with their true power, and when they are willing to assume responsibility for this, we will reclaim the power of birth and help move technology where it belongs—in the service of birthing women, not as their master.[13]

Okay, let's get this question out of the way. *Is a natural birth the only way to a peaceful birth?* The short answer is—drumroll, please—no, you do not have to have a natural birth in order to have a peaceful birth. It is just light-years easier to have a peaceful birth if it is natural.

Let's say you have a recipe for chocolate chip cookies, and I have a recipe for chocolate chip cookies. The ingredients may vary, the measurements may be different, but in the end we both get chocolate chip cookies that we equally enjoy. But there are basic ingredients you need in order to get a chocolate chip cookie. Flour, a liquid, a sweetener, something to make them rise a bit, and the chocolate chips.

While the exact ingredients and measurements may vary, and your recipe may actually have more ingredients and be more complicated than mine, the point is, you need the basics. To achieve a peaceful birth, this is what you need:

1. Faith and confidence in yourself.
2. A connection with your unborn baby.
3. A trusting, strong, respectful, autonomous relationship with your primary caregiver, if you choose to hire one at all.
4. A trusting, supportive environment.
5. A supportive, loving, faithful, experienced birth team, unless you are choosing to birth alone.

Now, you will notice that I didn't list a vaginal, C-section, medicated, natural, spontaneous or forced (induced), or a home or hospital delivery. The goal here is to improve the quality of the birth no matter the method or outcome. I am grateful to know and have been taught by women who have had or attended births that have been peaceful and empowering, yet still ended in a C-section, medicated birth, or even stillbirth.

Acquiring these ingredients for a peaceful birth is just more likely and plentifully found when you are planning a natural birth and/or out-of-hospital birth. That's not to say that if you choose to have intervention, like an epidural, induction or C-section, that you still can't employ all the ingredients of a peaceful birth. And if the unexpected is necessitated, like an unplanned C-section or stillbirth, you need those ingredients more than ever. If you have any other type of birth experience besides a natural, vaginal birth – whether it was of your choosing or not - you can still have a peaceful birth, it may just take more work. It's common for women to comment to natural birthers or home birthers, "Oh, you're so brave/strong, I could never do that." What they don't realize is that, for long-term outcomes and satisfaction, it's much easier to birth naturally and/or out of hospital than to follow the status quo. While a peaceful birth that is also a natural one requires a lot of preparation, shedding of old destructive beliefs, regaining of innate knowledge, and the literal hard, physical work during labor and birth, the benefits far outweigh the work it takes to get there.

There are lifelong health, emotional, and spiritual benefits to you, your child, and your family to birth the way nature designed it. It's much harder to say the same thing of an interventive, medicated birth. Much harder, but not impossible. If, ultimately, you decide that a medicated, induced, or surgical birth is the best route for you, in order to achieve that peaceful state, it's imperative you hire a caregiver you have a trusting, autonomous relationship with, then hire a doula who strives to keeps the atmosphere as normal and peaceful as possible, and meditate or do whatever you need to in order to stay in a peaceful mindset. Prepare as best you can, and enter in with confidence and faith in yourself.

I once had a client who was having her third baby. She very much wanted an intervention-free birth but felt her circumstances necessitated an induction. Her doctor supported her wishes to choose her induction method; Pitocin IV drip, Cervidil, or artificial rupture of her membranes (breaking her water). The day of the induction arrived and she was still undecided on how to proceed. She looked to me, her husband, and the nurse and asked us what we would do personally in this situation. I'm glad she directed her question at me first, as I believe my answer set the tone.

"Look, you know all the pros and cons to each induction method. It would be really unfair and manipulative of me to tell you what I'd do. You are the one who has to walk away with this experience under your belt, and I want you to be as powerful as possible throughout the labor and birth. This is a decision only you can make. You will make the right one."

Ultimately, she chose to have her water broken. She began contracting spontaneously soon thereafter and had a wonderful, natural, very low-intervention birth. She and her husband were on cloud nine about it.

My point is, even though it wasn't her ideal and she felt an induction was necessary, she still felt autonomous and empowered and walked away happy because everything that happened was her decision and her entire birth team respected and supported her. The fact that we refused to take away her power and decision making from her—even when she wanted us to—played a significant role in her positive and healthy experience.

Another client, who was having her second baby, felt very impressed that she needed to plan a C-section. She had been through my class series, hired me as her doula, and wanted a vaginal birth after Cesarian (VBAC), but just never felt peaceful about a vaginal birth. I made sure that she had covered all her bases about her decision to have a repeat Cesarean and I supported her decision to follow her gut. Then I helped her plan out as many details of the birth that she could have control over. She ended up having as peaceful and empowering a C-section as one can possibly have. She and her husband had nothing but good to say about the experience.

Another great example comes from Jonelle, my very good friend and colleague. Early on in her doula career, one of her client's births took an unexpected turn. Very quickly a Cesarean was decided on and the woman was put under general anesthesia. During the whole process, even when she was unconscious, Jonelle talked her through the surgery, step by step, all along reassuring and comforting her. She told her client, as she was unconscious, when the doctor was cutting, when the baby's head and body were out, that the baby was healthy and details of how the baby looked, and that she was safe. The anesthesiologist attempted to "enlighten" Jonelle by letting her know that her client couldn't hear her. Jonelle just smiled and continued whispering into her client's ear. After the birth, this new mom said to Jonelle, "I remember you saying she had a full head of brown hair." She went on to let Jonelle know just how vital her presence, support, and love aided her in putting the pieces of the labor and birth experience together and remembering it in a positive light.

Again, you don't need to have a natural or out-of-hospital birth in order to achieve a peaceful birth; you just may have more work to do to achieve it.

> We learn the lessons in life we are to learn two ways: either through obedience to natural laws or through suffering the consequences of not observing those laws . . . none of us consciously create the suffering we experience.
> —Karol Truman
> *Feelings Buried Alive Never Die*

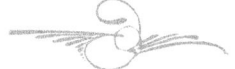

## What This Book Is, and What This Book Is Not

Before we move on, I want you to be clear on what exactly you can expect from this book. This book is:

1. Hope. There *is* a positive birth experience waiting out there for you. Without hope, what is the point of even trying to do anything? So hope is by far one of the most, if not the most important thing to have in birth—or in life for that matter.
2. A template of what is possible. When you are aware of your options and choices, suddenly you become free to explore your potential in birth.
3. Encouragement. When you are brought to the brink of what you think is your breaking point, it is invaluable to look up and have someone who has been in your

shoes say, "Yes, you *can* do it. Stay with it. You are so close." We all deserve that kind of encouragement, especially in the process of achieving a peaceful birth where we have so many naysayers and detractors.

This book is *not* a guarantee that your birth will unfold exactly how you want. *I* can't guarantee you anything just by offering you this book. No one can guarantee you a safe birth, a pain-free birth, or any other kind of birth, but *you* can choose to seek and create a peaceful birth, even if your outcome is different than your ideal.

I once asked one of my nurse friends, before she entered the profession, why she was choosing that route. I was happy to hear that job security, insurance coverage, and predictable hours were her second, third, and fourth reasons and not her first. Her first reason was that she wanted to be someone "on the inside" who could comfort and guide those who couldn't have a peaceful birth. She wanted to fly under the radar and change the fear-based hospital protocol from within. I assert that her belief—that not everyone can have a peaceful birth—is what is currently in the driver's seat of perpetuating our depressed birth economy in this and other countries.

By assuming that disasters happen and then looking for them, you will not only find them, but you will co-create them. There will never be a shortage of people there to pick up the pieces of a shattered birth experience; however, what we need is triple the amount of people working to help achieve peaceful birth experiences. You do more to prevent traumatic births by striving for your own peaceful birth and helping others achieve theirs.

# 2

## Limits and Possibilities
## Self-Test Pop Quiz

**L**et's pause a moment before you move on with the rest of the book. In order to progress and achieve your peaceful birth, I think it's vital you ponder and answer the following questions honestly. The truth is that we have been unconsciously programmed into thinking of birth in certain ways. This quiz can reveal just how much deprogramming you may need to undergo. Don't worry, there will be no poking, prodding, or large machinery involved in this deprogramming.

1. Are you afraid that if you achieve your peaceful birth, your friends, family, and social circle might ridicule you, belittle you, or reject you in some way? In other words, do you feel you'll lose your social support by making choices that defy your "tribal rules"? Do you fear being kicked out of or losing your standing in your "tribe"?
2. Growing up, were you told and believed that pregnancy and childbirth was a harrowing sacrifice that women were cursed with and you had to suffer as a form of payment to have your children and experience joy in them?
3. Do you or would you feel guilty for enjoying your birth experience in light of the fact that none of your family

and friends have?

4. Were you raised to believe that you don't question doctors or authority figures, and it's always best to just do as the doctor says?
5. Do you or did you grow up liking TV shows, movies or books where women never take responsibility and are always in the middle of a drama?
6. Are you always waiting for the "ball to drop"? Do you believe that life is always full of challenge and there will always be barriers to achieving what you want, preventing you from fulfilling your dreams?
7. Are you jealous of other women who have realized their desires in birth and parenting? Do you secretly resent them and discredit them behind their backs?
8. Do you admire women who have endured traumatic births, such as unplanned Cesareans, forceps/vacuum extractions, death or serious illness of their babies?
9. Have you had a negative birth experience, complained about it, blamed others, then did nothing the second time around to improve on it?
10. Have you ever used derogatory expressions like *earthy birthy, birth nazi,* or *freak* to describe other women's birth philosophies?
11. Do you use excuses like, "Well, if I had a husband/partner as good as yours," "It's too expensive," "Well, I've had a previous C-section, pre-eclampsia, inability to go into labor on my own, so I can't do X, Y, or Z"?
12. Do you like to tell your stories of victimization? On any level, would you secretly like the power, attention, and sympathy that telling a horror birth story would give you?
13. Do you feel like you could find the resources (money, caregiver, health, and support) to achieve your dream birth, but feel like you just don't have the energy, time, or courage to take the necessary steps to accomplish it?

Tally your results here

_____Yes          _____No

*If you answered no for 11–13 questions*

You have a high birth IQ. You can likely just move on to the next chapter without examining your birth philosophy in relation to achieving a peaceful birth.

*If you answered yes to 4 or 5 questions*

Subconsciously your risk of sabotaging yourself away from a peaceful birth is elevated. You have hang-ups, fears, or self-doubts you need to replace with surrendering, confidence, and faith in yourself and in the birth process. You are likely happy with life and yourself, but there isn't much you are "on fire" about. You want a peaceful birth, but don't know exactly what that means or why you want it.

*If you answered yes to 6 or 7 questions*

You live by the creed, "Two steps forward, one step back," so you never really make large steps toward your goals. You find it difficult to accept that your dream birth is within your reach. It is my observation that this is where about half of American women are.

*If you answered yes to 8 or more questions*

You are already on a very dramatic path in your pregnancy and it looks like you'll likely end up with a birth you don't want unless you start implementing mental shifts soon—like today. You feel trapped, with little to no hope. It is of the utmost importance you claim your pregnancy and birth *now!* Stop letting others make your decisions. Admitting that you espouse negative and false beliefs about yourself, pregnancy, birth, and motherhood on a subconscious level might be hard, but by replacing them with true and positive beliefs, you can break this cycle gracefully.

So are your beliefs true or false? Helping or hurting?

To a large extent, your birth is going to reflect your beliefs not only about birth, but also about yourself, your parenting abilities, your relationships, and your place in your tribe and the world.

> The power and intensity of your contractions cannot be stronger than you, because it is you.
> —Anonymous

Whether your beliefs are true or false, hurtful or helpful, they are very real to you right now. I encourage you to take all your beliefs about births and make sure they are true and helpful. If they aren't, you have the power to change them *right now.*

Changing your beliefs begins by defining and being specific about what you want. As soon as you define what you want, all your beliefs, whether they are helpful or hurtful to your goal, will surface. Whatever is a hindrance needs to be written down, and then you need to verbalize the reverse of that belief and internalize it.

This is actually easier than you think. In fact, for most people, it's easier than you want it to be. Sometimes an answer is so simple and easy that we don't give it credit and pass right over it. The hard part is letting go of your false beliefs and stepping into something that you have previously not explored.

> Within you right now is the power to do things you never dreamed possible. This power becomes available to you just as you can change your beliefs.
> —Maxwell Maltz

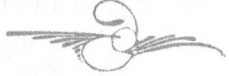

## Rejecting vs. Embracing the Truths That Find You

A while ago I was talking with a friend of a friend. This woman had numerous wonderful qualities about her, many I aspire to develop, but I left our conversation tempted to label her quite the Debbie Downer.

This woman had just had her third "horror story" birth experience, and while she was very intelligent, generous and charitable, she had the art of dismissal down to a science. Any positive thing I had to say about pregnancy, birth, and breast-feeding—shoot, come to think of it, even sex—with the exception of saying anything positive about the actual baby, I was met with a counter comment whenever I spoke glowingly of the birth year. That conversation, and dare I say potential friendship, had a very short shelf life

I don't think she was doing it on a conscious level. I think if someone had recorded the conversation, she'd be a little off-put by her own comments. But on an unconscious level, she rejected everything that would lead her to a peaceful birth. She was self-sabotaging.

At one point I told her about this amazing birth I attended. I went on and on about how the mom moved so gracefully through her birth and responded to her sensations with acceptance and love. How both the mom and dad walked away with this overwhelming sense of power and connectivity that they described it as the best drug trip they've ever had.

This woman cut me off and said, "I've known women who have had similar births and have walked away absolutely hating it. They'd never do it again."

What was I going to say to that? I knew her as an honest person, so I trusted she wasn't lying just to make a point. But then I realized that while she may have known women who had birthed in similar settings and circumstances, with the same people, via the same "route" (i.e., natural birth, medicated or surgical birth), they had not birthed *in peace* like this couple had; had they done so there's no way they could have walked away unhappy. In pondering this, I also remembered, via conversations with our mutual friend, how many years this lady had been struggling with depression. I realized that her frequent bouts with misery likely colored the lens through which she experienced our conversation – so that she missed the distinction between a mere natural birth and the peaceful birth I was describing.

When we dismiss other's pregnancy, birth, and postpartum experiences because not everyone walks away from them with a positive, empowering feeling, we get to be right. And we also get the validation and attention from telling our "horror birth story." By rejecting what might be possible for ourselves—that peaceful, graceful, beautiful birth experience—we deny ourselves even the slightest chance of achieving it.

When a woman extols the virtues of her pregnancy, birth, and postpartum experience, do you sit back in superior silent judgment or disapproval? Good. Pay attention to that, because now you know you have a negative belief system that you use unconsciously to base your decisions on, and admitting it is the first step.

*When you judge another, you do not define them, you define yourself.*
—Wayne Dyer

Truth be told, not one way of birthing is going to work for everyone. Vaginal birth isn't going to work for everyone, natural birth isn't, and Cesarean isn't. No one caregiver is going to work for everyone. No one birthplace is going to meet everyone's needs. But only you will know what will work for you. You are the expert on you. No one else. And because you are the expert on you, you are the expert on the baby inside of you. You are not separate. Instead of denying what it possible for yourself so that you can be right, open your heart and ask yourself, why not me?

All the women and couples I know who have had peaceful births have sought out others who have themselves birthed joyously, and have opened themselves up to a new (at least new to them) way of thinking, have invested time, energy, and money into learning all they can and have been happy they have done it, even if their birth didn't go according to plan.

Don't discount out of hand people's experiences or new approaches, but instead explore and internalize them, see if they resonate with you.

For example, years ago I ran into a friend and her young children at the park accompanied by one of her friends. Once her friend found out I was a doula, she went on and on about how she wished she could have a doula, but that she'd had a previous Cesarean and she believed her doctors when they told her she would always have Cesareans. She was advised to have only one or two more children. She told me about just how sad she was over the whole ordeal. She had always wanted a big family, she said, and wanted nice birth experiences, but it just wasn't in the cards for her. She was just grateful for the one or two more children she could have and for the one she had now. She gave me every roadblock in the book. You name it, she was stuck. This was her lot in life and she had finally come to terms with it, she said, even though it pained her to.

What I was actually doing at the park that day was waiting to meet up with my mom's group for our weekly park day. I said little to this new acquaintance as she was recounting her circumstances to me, keeping in mind that I hadn't even asked about her birthing experiences, but I was happy to listen. In the back of my head, I knew the best thing for this woman was to not hear anything from me, but to hear from someone who had once been in her heavy, lonely shoes. One of the moms in the group, Olivia we'll call her, I knew was coming in just a few minutes. Olivia had actually overcome the same obstacles this new acquaintance lamented about, and had had multiple, incredible VBACs.

Olivia showed up and I introduced the two, briefly stating that our new friend shared a similar birth experience as she had with her first birth. "Oh really?" Olivia asked excitedly. Olivia innocently assumed that our new friend was desirous to achieve a beautiful VBAC as well. Immediately Olivia started offering this woman hope and encouragement. As she spoke, our new friend interjected, repeating the sad news that she had told me, but Olivia just continued on, knowing that more likely than not, our new friend might feel inspired.

"Well, what if I told you that what you were told isn't true?" Olivia probed.

Our new friend was thrown off a bit. I could tell no one had ever challenged her on her beliefs, "What do you mean?" she asked.

"Well, it sounds like we had our C-sections for the same reasons. I've since had three incredible VBAC's. Do you want a VBAC?" Olivia probed.

I was excited. I had actually seen similar scenarios play out with phenomenal results. But what did our new friend do with this door that had just been opened? She closed it. Actually, she slammed it. With a firm grip on the handle, and a forced smile on her face, she quietly and decidedly closed the door. She didn't ask who Olivia's caregiver was, her birthplace, or what she had done to prepare. Nothing that would indicate that an angel had just landed in her lap and told her that all she said she wanted, she could actually achieve.

Are you getting the picture? Whatever the reasons you have accepted—fear, self-doubt, self-loathing, complacency—we can deny ourselves the experience, and sometimes even the children, we say we want.

Women often want to know what one book or item they can get that will give them the greatest odds of achieving their dream births. I tell them that, if nothing else, hire a great doula. Not your mom or your sister, not your massage therapist friend who thinks she can navigate the unfamiliar hospital and labor territory, but a trained, great doula.

Some complain that insurance doesn't cover them, or that a doula is expensive. Yes, a doula will ask to be compensated in some way. She has paid for trainings, is going to be on call, has to find on-call childcare and be gone an undetermined amount of time, possibly getting no food or sleep and getting thrown up on. Are you going to invest and increase your odds of a peaceful birth, for which there are no do-overs, or are you going to cross your fingers and wing it, all in the name of saving some money? What's more expensive: a doula, or a birth experience you didn't want and possible negative health effects?

Look around. Listen. Ask. Seek. Your peaceful birth isn't going to happen by winging it. Trust me, I've doulaed for plenty of people who tried to wing it the first time around and then realized they should have been more careful.

> Deep listening is miraculous for both listener and speaker. When someone receives us with open-hearted, non-judging, intensely interested listening, our spirits expand.
> —Sue Patton Theole

## Storytelling:
## Realizing What You Are Learning and Teaching

*The Birth of Cedar Olivia Part 1: The Dress Rehearsal*
*All right, here we go. I'd been preparing for this birth with Hypnobabies, and part of that program involves visualizing the details of your birth. I chose to visualize a Friday birth between the hours of 1 a.m. and 6 a.m. Yeah, I don't play around. I threw down the gauntlet.*

*On Friday, three days past my "guess date," at*

approximately 1 p.m. (okay, so it didn't work perfectly), I had a gush of fluid while standing in the kitchen. I was home alone. The fluid was clear. But it did not continue to leak like it had during Norah's birth. I thought perhaps Cedar's head had sealed it since the baby was already very low. My pressure waves (Hypnobabies lingo for contractions) began immediately and were about 3–4 minutes apart. I listened to Cedar using a doppler and she sounded great. I waited an hour and then called Scott to come home. The waves continued and I listened to a couple of Hypnobabies scripts on my iPod. Everything was very relaxed and manageable. I called my sister and told her to come when she wanted to.

As things continued, I noticed that I was very much in my head. In other words, I was thinking too much. I was trying to doula myself (this laboring mom is a doula), and the waves were spacing out. In an effort to get my mind elsewhere, I asked if we could play Pass the Pigs, a game that always makes me laugh. Except for one stellar Leaning Jowler, I tossed a terrible game (Scott won), but I laughed so hard. Then we thought maybe we should go out to eat. So we went for Mexican where I ate a ton of food and had great pressure waves.

When we returned home, it felt like Cedar had spun from ROA (right occiput anterior, baby's back against mom's abdomen) to a posterior (baby's back against mom's back) position. Pressure waves were spacing again. We decided to try the birth tub. The water should either stop things or intensify them.

Let me interject here that the La Bassine birth tub rocks! It was deep and roomy. The floor inflates making it very comfortable and it has internal handles. I hopped in. It felt marvelous. And, the waves spaced even farther. But it was nice. Scott was playing the guitar and singing some Iron and Wine. Noelle had gone to bed. It was an intimate and sweet time. I got out of the tub and Scott got in. His back was sore so he had some therapeutic time in the water. Then we went to bed. Okay, I admit I went to bed utterly deflated.

When I woke the next morning, I felt embarrassed and discouraged. As a doula, I should have known if I was in "real" labor. Good thing Noelle is a counselor since I needed some emotional processing (over chocolate muffins) Saturday morning. Scott and I decided to spend the day watching movies, snuggling, and eating yummy food. I cried several times through the day. Hindsight: it was really nice to have a dress rehearsal and from the intensity of many of the waves, it was "real" labor. It was spinning the baby into position. Maybe it was changing my cervix some. More importantly, it gave me some warning that I needed to stop thinking like a doula and let my intuition take the reins. I wasn't sure how I was going to do that though.

Saturday night, as Scott was rubbing some pressure points on my lower legs, I watched my belly as Cedar spun to LOA (left occiput anterior)–the best position for beginning birth.

Now we were ready.

The Birth of Cedar Olivia Part 2: Places, Everybody

Where was I? Oh yes, utterly deflated. Late Saturday night, we went to Publix to buy groceries. I had clipped all the coupons already so I had to go. Right, coupon moms? Then I stayed up too late and went to sleep listening to a Hypnobabies script. During the night, I felt pressure waves come and go but ignored them. At 6 a.m., I thought I might time a couple—10 minutes apart. No big deal then. I listened to another script. Around 7:45, Scott brought a warm rice sock and turned on some Fleet Foxes. What a nice way to wake.

At 9 a.m., it was like someone flipped a switch. I was making breakfast when the pressure waves went from 10 minutes apart to a very serious 3 minutes apart. The energy changed and I told Scott I was having a baby today. I managed to eat my eggs and toast while standing and rocking. Again, I noticed how much I was thinking like a doula. What position should I take? Should Scott shift me? What about belly-lifting? Do I need to do the rotisserie? Argh, the voice in my head!

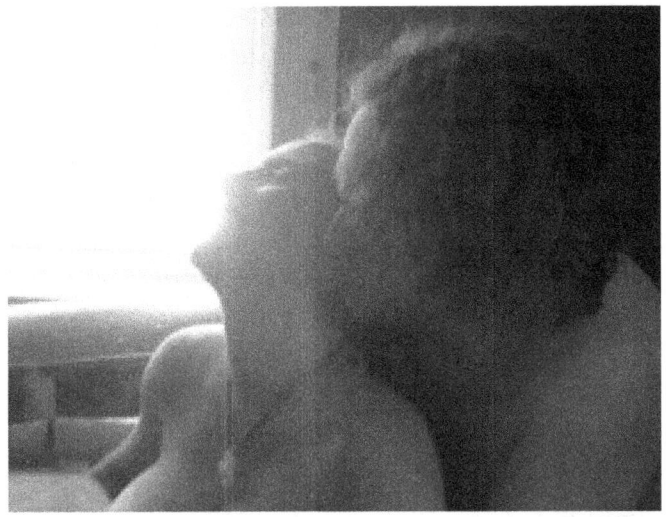

Then, without thinking, with the next pressure wave, I began reciting T.S. Eliot's "The Love Song of J. Alfred Prufrock." Yes, a poem about a balding man's mid-life crisis. Yes, that is the focal point I chose folks. Not a nice Psalm. Not a beautiful song. Not even a poet like Neruda or Rilke. I could recite to line 22 ("curled once about the house, and fell asleep") before the wave ended. I did not feel pain just an intense squeezing sensation.

At 10:35 a.m., Scott wrote in the birth log that I said a horrible curse word. Friends–brace yourself. At the end of a pressure wave during which I forgot the words to my poem, I said "Dad-gum." Time to get into the birth tub. Ah, the birth tub. Bliss. I could drape over the sides and flip my Hypnobabies light switch to "off."

Using hypnosis, I totally kicked transition's butt. Oh yeah. Smiling and relaxing, this birth was a piece of cake. Until at 1 p.m., I swore again. Scott notes that I said "Yowzers." I should interject that Cedar was sounding beautiful. She was actively involved and had a great heart rate the whole time. Never gave us a worry.

I began feeling a little pushy. I was really looking forward to pushing. My firstborn, Norah, was so easy-breezy to push (although her 32 hours of labor was challenging). I pushed Norah out in 20-something minutes with barely a sound. Ah, but Cedar. My first tentative push with Cedar told me something was different. And I began to fear. Fear+birth=pain. What was I afraid of? Well the doula brain was happy to rush back into high gear and tell me. I was afraid of a posterior baby. A nuchal hand. Tearing. Having to transport for suturing. Shut up, thinking brain!

Scott got into the tub at 1:20 and I tried pushing a few times while standing up. Then squatting. Both were overwhelming in sensation. I birthed Norah while squatting and I was barely aware of her descent. In fact, she took all of us by surprise when she tumbled out in between contractions.

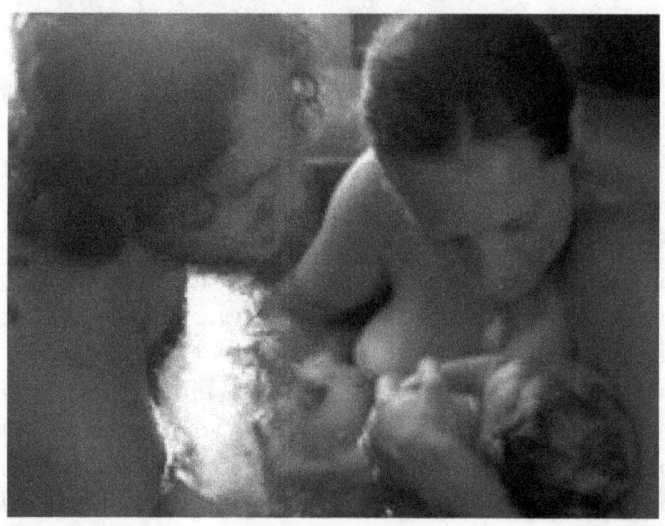

Cedar. Oh Cedar. First to present was the bag of waters–yep, still intact. I felt it with my hand and it was so hard. Until it broke–nice gush of clear fluid. Then, I felt Cedar descending like a freight train. I was on my knees but moved to a knee-crouch kind of position. Really, I think I was crouched because I was contemplating jumping out of the tub and just running away. Scott applied counter pressure to my perineum. I put pressure on my front and around the head. Wow, the sensations were incredible; and not incredible like orgasmic birth incredible. Nope, none of that. Scott said something later about feeling the energy and power of my uterus. He said birth should be an Olympic sport because of that powerful muscle.

Cedar was born at 2:18. Scott caught her and brought her to the surface. She was not posterior. No nuchal hand. And I did not tear. On my chest, I rubbed her and snuggled her. She looked so healthy. And she was. I didn't want to look to see if she was a girl or boy. That took some time.

After the placenta came, Scott clamped and cut the cord. No one noted the time but I know Cedar was already nursing by then. We got out of the tub. I drank some OJ. We examined Cedar (heart rate, respiration, temp, etc). Unfortunately, my bleeding was a bit heavy and my uterus was not clamping down as well as it could have. So I got a shot of Pitocin, took some herbs, and had lots of "fun" fundal massage to get my uterus to contract. What moron decided to call it "massage" anyway?

Cedar weighed in at 8 lbs 10 oz and was 21 inches long.

Then we all went to bed. And I pretty much stayed there for five days. Snuggling and nursing and being visited by lovely family and friends. And sweet midwives-to-be Carey and Crystal picked up my placenta the next day and encapsulated it for me. I also discovered how wonderful coconut water is for restoring electrolytes.

—Julie, inexplicableways.com

My paternal grandmother, who always had her wits about her, recounted with detail in her last years, all four of her births to me. I was so struck by just how real the emotion of the births still were to her. She reflected the joy she felt and was still as angry as she likely was the day of the events about the disappointments when she was retelling those stories. Sadly, I didn't write the experiences down when she told them to me. Since I didn't and don't want to do her injustice, I asked her daughter (my Aunt Carla) to give us an account of those experiences. As you read them, I want you to think of your own grandmother or other relative whom you love, and ask yourself what kind of birth experiences they had, and ponder how those experiences shaped who they are, who your parents are and who you are, because births have a generational ripple effect.

> Jerrold was born August 6, 1931, in the hospital located in St. George, Utah. Mother said that she had a long hard labor with him and when, after pushing and pushing and bearing down for all she was worth, the doctor reached into the birth canal and literally pulled Jerrold out with forceps! When Mother at last was able to hold Jerrold for the first time she was dismayed to see how bruised his head was—she could see the indentation marks the forceps left on his head. She also said that his head was shaped like an egg from being in the birth canal so long. It took awhile before his head resumed its normal shape. Jerrold was a large baby and weighed around 10 pounds.

This was my father's birth. When I first heard this story I was struck by the fact that when, although very rarely, my dad would get angry, he would get these rings of red inflammation on both sides of his head. When I found out he was a forceps baby, this explained the rings, not to mention it broke my heart.

> Before I [Carla] was born, Mother and Dad's finances did not allow for me to be born in the hospital in St. George and so they made arrangements for the doctor to come to their home to attend Mother—in fact they paid him in advance to do this. My dad had waited as long as he could for me to be born but he could wait no longer as he had to deliver the mail to the Arizona Strip. Well, as I was ready to make my grand entrance, the doctor took off for Las Vegas to have a good time! That left my dad's mother to deliver me. She had never delivered a baby before and was terribly nervous and upset. Mother had a long labor with me and she told me later that she squatted by the side of the bed and bore down for all she was worth but to no avail. She finally got back on the bed (because Grandma made her!) and then she pushed and pushed and pulled and pulled on Grandma's arms until Grandma didn't have any more strength to help her. Without asking Mother if

it was okay, Grandma asked Grandpa and my dad's oldest brother to come and let my mother pull on their arms as she pushed and bore down to deliver me. My mother was not happy having Grandpa and her brother-in-law there. She was in fact quite angry to have them in the same room. Grandma was scared and although the hour was very late she decided to go next door to ask her neighbor to come and help. By then, Mother was so mad that she gave one good hard push and bore down for all she was worth and as Grandma arrived with Mrs. Seegmiller, I decided to make my arrival. Mother told me that my grandmother delivered me. After the excitement was all over, it was after midnight and Mrs. Seegmiller asked if anyone knew what time I'd been born. My mother spoke up and said, "Put down that she was born before midnight—I want her born in June, not July!" So, it was entered on my birth certificate that I was born before midnight, June 30, 1934. My dad paid Mrs. Seegmiller for her services with a load of wood that was worth $15.00.

    Mother said that my brother Michael's birth was a joy! By then, my dad had a good paying job and arrangements were made ahead of time for my mother to go to a "confinement home" in Carson City, Nevada. We were living in Gold Hill, Nevada, at that time, which is about half an hour drive away from Carson City. When Mother felt that it was about time for the baby to be born, she was in the process of making a huge pot of chili. When I asked her why she was making so much she told me that she was ready to have a baby and she wanted to make sure we had something to eat while she was gone. When I heard she was going to have a baby, I said, "Oh, can I be the first to tell Daddy?" (I've never lived that remark down and have always been known to be quite naive.) Mother said that she was treated so very kindly at this "confinement home" and she was relaxed and her delivery was easy. Michael was born February 21, 1942. Mother stayed at this place for 10 days before she came home with Michael— she said it was like she had been on a vacation.

    Well, Shelby was a different story! We were living in

Las Vegas, Nevada, when Mother was ready to deliver him. Arrangements had already been made for her to go to the Las Vegas Hospital for the delivery and that Dr. Hardy would be the attending physician. When Mother felt it was time to go to the hospital, her labor pains were harder than usual, and when she got to the hospital she learned that Dr. Hardy could not be reached and oh! goodness, but Mother was mad! Dad was with her and he tried to calm her down. The attending nurse said she'd never delivered a baby before and told Mother to wait to have the baby until Dr. Hardy could get there! That remark did not help Mother! It just made her all the more upset! By then, she was on the gurney and was ready to have this baby no matter what the nurse said! The nurse tried to push Mother's knees together to prevent her from bearing down. Mother was so angry that she shoved the nurse aside and told my Dad to catch the baby 'cause it was coming now! So, Dad delivered my little brother and the nurse calmed down enough to tie the cord. Shelby was born October 6, 1943.

Our birth experiences stay with us. We will remember them for the rest of our lives. I feel for my mother's and grandmother's generation, who had to deal with whatever birth traumas they had alone and invalidated, for the most part. It was not common to talk about birth in our grandmother's generation, and certainly it was taboo to speak of the very traumatic parts that were inflicted on women and babies. I'm grateful to my grandmother for being so open and honest with her experiences. And I am grateful she had some birth experiences that allowed her to see the beauty of birth and the depth of her strength. She was a strong and beautiful lady.

Birth experiences can also stay with our babies. Whether it's something overtly or subtly physical, like my dad's red rings on his face, or the emotional effects of how they were treated antenatally or during and after birth, these experiences can stay with our babies, too. As Bruce Lipton points out in his book *The Biology of Belief*:

> Stress hormones prepare the body to engage in a protection response. Once these maternal signals enter

the bloodstream, they affect the same target tissues and organs in the fetus as they did in the mother. In stressful environments, fetal blood preferentially flows to the muscles and hindbrain, providing nutritional requirements needed by the arms and legs and by the region of the brain responsible for life saving reflex behavior. In supporting the function of the protection related systems, blood flow is shunted from the viscera organs and stress hormones suppress forebrain function. . . . When passing through the placenta, the hormones of a mother experiencing chronic stress will profoundly alter the distribution of blood flow in her fetus and change the character of her developing child's physiology.[14]

In layman's terms, when you're stressed, your baby's stressed. When you're at peace, your baby is at peace. Stress is destructive, and peace promotes growth. Lipton continues:

Information acquired from the parents' perception of their environment transits the placenta and primes the prenate's physiology, preparing it to more effectively deal with future exigencies that will be encountered after birth. Nature is simply preparing that child to best survive in that environment. However, armed with the latest science, parents now have a choice. They can carefully reprogram their limiting beliefs about life before they bring a child into their world.[15]

Many women have no problem accepting the notion that their emotional and mental state shapes their unborn baby's temperament, and in fact, many cultures still have many old wives tales (that are being backed up by science such as Lipton's) that dictate better treatment of pregnant women to ensure the best possible outcome for the baby. But for some reason, our society seems to think that the well-being and development of the unborn baby is somehow put on hold during the labor and birth process. As if stress, isolation, cruelty, fear, and even pain have no short- or long-term effects on babies who experience those things during labor and birth. This approach extends into the early postpartum period where babies have bright lights shined in their eyes, cold temperatures to acclimate to, and loud and unwelcoming noises to filter out. Then they are routinely separated from their most intimate source, their mother, and poked, prodded, and roughly handled. And then we expect them to nurse with ease and bond and be happy? The way babies are routinely handled in the PABC, and have been for over a century, stresses them and places them at risk of emotional and physical shut down.

A traumatized mother/baby pair is not exactly the best foot to start off with for parents. Add to that a possibly traumatized father as well, and you've got yourself a recipe for quite a hard time.

I want to emphasize that should you and/or your baby experience a less than peaceful birth and postpartum experience, you are not doomed to failure and a lifetime of pain associated with those memories. In fact, it's those parents and babies who need the most attention and care. This is one reason why I so highly recommend birth and postpartum doula care, babymooning, and participation in good support groups that promote peaceful birth and parenting experiences. Lipton also recommends seeking out healing through energy work, of which I have personal experience with and recommend highly as well.

The following is a birth story from one of my clients, and I hope that it gives you some tools to address any pain you have, or may have, and also recover and heal.

> Rosy's third birth
> I knew the moment I saw that second pink line appearing on the pregnancy test that I wanted an unmedicated birth. This would be my third child and I felt finally ready to experience the kind of birth I had always dreamed about. For as long as I can remember, I have been drawn to birth stories. I love the intensity, the humility, the strength, and just the raw beauty of it all. It has always made me feel proud to be a woman and excited that I might possess the strength to walk through that shadow of death to bring a child into the world.
>
> *I became pregnant with my first child in the middle of nursing school. The semester I found out, we happened to be studying a maternal newborn class. I felt torn as I went to my weekly clinical on the Labor and Delivery floor.*

Woman after woman came into the hospital in severe pain only to have it all be taken away with a little (or very large) shot in her back. My nerves got to me, and I started to doubt that I could endure the pain naturally. Those doubts led to me getting an epidural when I was just dilated to a 3 and feeling the intensity. I will be honest that my epidural went as smooth as can be. It seemed to take the edge off, and I happily labored, even feeling the urge to push! Afterward I thought, "Well this is the way to go. Why would anyone want to go through all that pain?"

This thinking led me to receive an epidural with my second child less than two years later. I was dilated to a 6 and doing pretty well when the nurse started pestering me about getting an epidural. I felt like I was fine, but agreed that I didn't want to "miss the window." One minute after I received my injection I felt completely paralyzed. I had absolutely no feeling from the waist down. Something did not feel right, and I began to panic. The anesthesiologist turned the epidural dosage down, and assured me everything was just fine. I continued to labor, never feeling a thing. When it came time to push, all I could do was make pushing faces to appease the nurses. They ended up pushing down on my abdomen to help me birth my baby boy.

Six hours postpartum I hemorrhaged. I became very unstable and began passing out from the loss of blood. The medical team acted quickly and were able to stop the bleeding. I still had absolutely no feeling below the waist, and this continued until 13 hours after birth when I was finally able to wiggle my toes. I thought a lot about birth for the next few months and felt disturbed with the idea of completely numbing/paralyzing a woman's body during such a defining experience, one in which it was perfectly created for. I promised myself that I would not miss out again.

From the moment I found out that I was pregnant for a third time, I began preparing. Over the next nine months, I read books about natural birth, chose a certified nurse midwife, hired a doula, and attended birth classes with my husband, Pascal. We felt prepared and were convinced that we would have a beautiful experience this time around.

My due date was November 24. My two previous babies came exactly one week early, so when my CNM, Laurie, told me "any day now" at 37 weeks, I believed her. Dilated to a 4 and 70 percent effaced, my due date came and went. I grew more and more frustrated with each appointment with all the pressure to be induced. I really wanted to begin labor on my own and truly felt that my body would do just that when it was good and ready. I agreed to set an induction date 10 days post due, but had a prayer that it wouldn't have to come to that. In the meantime I focused on submitting to the process and allowing myself to be taught.

December 2, eight days over my due date, I began labor on my own. I labored at home for as long as possible in the tub with Pascal and my doula, Amy, by my side. I felt great. The contractions were painful but bearable, and my confidence grew that I really could achieve my goal of an unmedicated birth.

After about six hours of labor, we decided to head to the hospital. There, the nurse checked me—dilated to a 7 and 90 percent effaced! The pain was getting more and more intense and I headed for the bathtub.

The next few hours of labor were unimaginable. I had never felt pain like that. Each contraction was so powerful and humbling. It was amazing feeling my body work and progress naturally. I felt beautiful, feminine, and strong. There were moments I felt like I might lose control and just start screaming (or running), but through my strength, knowledge and support I had I was able to focus and endure.

After 12 hours of labor, I finally felt the urge to push. Wow! It was a very out-of-body experience for me. The pain and sensation are indescribable. There was something very primal about it, and I felt connected to every mother in nature. I was spiritually changed as our little girl entered the world.

Oh the joy! I did it! The birth was everything I had hoped for. I was so happy that it was all over (or so I thought) and that I would now be able to just hold and enjoy my baby girl.

*Our birth plan detailed that we wanted a good hour with our babe before the medical team intervened. I had often heard mothers talk about how wonderful and rewarding it is to just hold and bond with their little one after such grueling and hard work, so I had plans to do just that. The staff respected my wishes, and I held my baby while Laurie started to stitch my small tear.*

*But just five minutes after the birth my midwife became worried about my bleeding. My fundus (top of uterus) felt firm, so she couldn't figure out why I was continuing to lose blood. Everything became a whirlwind and the feeling of panic set in the room. My baby was taken away from me and the medical staff began pushing and prodding trying to find the source of the bleeding. Each push and "massage of the fundus" brought so much pain. I was still unmedicated and very overwhelmed with the whole birth experience I had just been through. I wanted relief; this pain was so much worse than labor and birth.*

*At least three times I screamed for my midwife to stop as she and the nurse would simultaneously inspect my uterus. She would reach up my vagina trying to feel my uterus for a laceration while the nurse would push down on my abdomen for Laurie to get a better feel.*

*I quickly felt the transition of person to patient. I no longer had a voice. I pleaded multiple times for them to stop and give me a breather, but to no avail. Even though I was stable, they were in their "save her life" mode and continued on as if I were in trouble anyway. Amy stayed by my side and held my hand trying to help me focus and breathe through the pain. I couldn't. I was not prepared for anything like this. I had spent the past nine months preparing for the beautiful experience I had just had, and I never thought that I would hemorrhage again. At this point my blood pressure was normal and though I blacked out a* few times from the pain of all the prodding and hands up inside me, my vitals remained stable, which is why I could not understand why all the panic and force.

My body began to tremble. I was going into shock, and I was freezing! I begged to get in the tub or for a warm blanket. I felt sure that if they would just give me 30 seconds to relax and focus, my body would do what it needed to.

But it was too late. My voice wasn't heard. From my years working as a nurse I could recognize that look on their faces. It was the look of procedures, interventions, and checklists. We were in separate worlds. They now viewed the problem at hand, not the person in front of them. They couldn't see me or hear me. They were referring to their books and training, and listening to the patient was not part of that training.

I still have horrible images of all the trauma. One of the most vivid is a point after my bleeding had slowed significantly and there was no more immediate medical issues where I had six tools up inside me tightly clamped to my uterus. I could sense that my CNM felt overwhelmed and maybe a little under experienced as she jumped from task to task. She left the room to get something or find someone and she left the clamps in me dangling from the hospital bed for what seemed like an eternity. I pleaded for somebody to hold them up and relieve the pull, but nobody but my CNM could touch the clamps and break sterile field. It was horrible. I felt such a frustration and was desperate to be heard. Finally, an IV was started for them to administer Pitocin intravenously. I had already received several intramuscular medications and now with the IV they decided to give me some pain medicine. This brought some relief and a lot of bitterness that it had taken so long.

The clamps remained inside of me while we waited for an OB to come give a second opinion. I continued a minimal, normal bleed. Looking back, I realize now that the bleeding was never a huge risk. It was the fact that they could not find the source of the bleeding. It was a panic of what could happen not what was really happening.

The OB came into the room and brought with him his knowledge and many years of experience a sense of calmness. He explained that I was among the few women whose uterus contracted on the top, but not along the bottom. This explained why my fundus felt firm, but yet, I continued to bleed. I was so relieved to have all the trauma and panic stop. I felt an air of defensiveness in the room as the medical team cleaned up. I was overwhelmed and crushed that my awesome birth experience had been followed by so much awfulness.

I didn't feel like I was ready to hold the baby quite yet. I felt removed and in shock with what had just happened for a solid hour and a half. At this moment, my doula, Amy, gave me a gift that I will forever be grateful. She validated me. She laid her cheek against mine and began to cry. I had such a powerful surge of emotion and I wept. Through her tears touching my face I felt an understanding. It was as if she was saying "I was there. I saw it. I'm sorry. I love you." She and Pascal stayed in the room and let me talk. They didn't try to justify or explain the interventions. They just heard me.

That night I didn't want to talk about either experience at all. I was having a hard time separating the two events. One was beautiful beyond belief and the other was horrible. Early that next morning and after a sleepless night, Pascal and I rehashed the events. He was so touched by the birth. He loved watching my strength and felt like it had changed him. I could feel how much our love had grown in just 24 hours. We talked for hours and I slowly began to remember the greatness of the birth.

Through a lot of love, prayer, support, and forgiveness I have felt the healing process take its course. I do not blame the medical team for seeing a problem and acting quickly. That is what they are trained to do. I just wish they had been trained to handle it with more compassion and care, and that they had listened to me! Regardless, I am truly grateful for the experience. I learned a lot about myself that day. I found an innate strength that I did not know I possessed. I was changed as only birth

*can change you. I am now more assertive, more powerful, more loving, more humble, more spiritual, and definitely more compassionate toward others. I will forever listen to what others are saying, especially in my role as a nurse. Do I wish I could go back and bypass all the trauma? Probably. But it's mine. And I love it.*
    —Roxy, mother of three

I pray that women today are seeking to heal their traumatic birth experiences, for themselves and their children, so that they can be liberated from that pain. Because even though we cannot change the events of the past, we can change how they shape us. Healing the pain of negative birth experiences can happen, and we can move forward and remember the experience without reliving the pain. But wouldn't we all be better off as women, mothers, and as a society if we didn't experience birth trauma in the first place? And wouldn't our babies be better off? I think that peaceful births in and of themselves would create more peace in this world than any treaty or alliance ever could.

How we birth our babies does matter, it is vitally important. And if you and/or your baby has experienced trauma or violation during a birth, it matters that you heal from it. Sometimes I'll meet with a second- or third-time parent, and if they've had a bad birth experience they'll use words like:

> *They made me.*
> *I had no choice.*
> *I had to block it out.*
> *They wouldn't move their hands when I told them to.*
> *I was screaming inside.*
> *I was scared to death.*
> *I wanted to cry and yell.*
> *I was forced.*

These expressions rend my heart. These are the words rape victims use to describe their experience. Anger, force, manipulation, coercion, and physical violations should never ever be a part of bringing life into this world. Ever. Even very subtle occurrences can have an effect.

One of the most common manipulative statements used in birth is "Well, if it were my wife, I'd do XYZ." I think that is terrible. It's not based on fact at all. To have a person in a position of authority tell you what he or she would do in efforts to try to sway your decision is unethical. The implication is that if you decide contrary to what the "authority" would do, you're being irresponsible.

Another one that drives nuts is "Get angry at your baby, push him out." What?! The first time I heard someone say that to a woman I was so incredibly bothered. Angry at your unborn baby? For what? Existing? Being exactly where the mother and father put him? Yes, that's exactly the energy needed to motivate a woman or her unborn to do the hard work of birthing and then love the baby she was just angry at. Not to mention how heartbreaking that those were the emotions communicated to the baby as he was making his entrance into the world. Talk about some negative imprinting. It's sad, and quite telling of our society's psyche, that referencing anger is the only way many birth professionals know how to communicate to a woman the energy she needs to push a baby out. No wonder there are organizations created to help women and men heal from birth experiences. We need them.

Those are just two minor examples of common situations, but my point is that there is always a way to treat people with compassion and love, no matter the situation, even in an emergency. It is needed *especially* in an emergency.

Because our society doesn't adequately recognize the post-traumatic stress after bad birth experiences, women and couples are sent on a downward spiral, not understanding why they are so angry, sad, fearful, and hurt.

> *Then suddenly the floodgates open. But these feelings are complicated. The woman feels bound to be grateful to the professionals who helped her deliver her baby, especially if the baby was perceived to be at risk, and yet these are the very people you feel have violated you. . . . This is not postnatal depression. These women have their birth experience going round and round in their heads like video on a loop. They can't switch it off. They are constantly reliving the trauma but rarely getting continuing*

support to deal with it. We need to find out what is most useful to women in this situation and what makes them feel worse. Then we can provide effective, individually-tailored support.
—Shiela Kitzinger, birth advocate and author

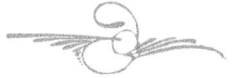

# What's Most Important: Reworking Our PABC Mantra

When a birth outcome is less than optimal or is otherwise not what the woman or couple has planned, most people, including the new parents, repeat the mantra (Sanskrit for "mind tool"), "The most important thing is that the baby is healthy."

That remark is about as comforting to me as nails on a chalkboard. It's not that I disagree—not completely, anyway. That remark bothers me so much because it's self-serving. It's what we say to make ourselves temporarily feel better, hoping that if we repeat it enough it'll actually make us feel better. But no one likes to talk about the very large, bright pink, very ugly, stinky, and ill-tempered elephant in the room.

Many people, especially those in the working within the PABC, will often try to make a very impassioned, fearful case that you can either have a live baby *or* a peaceful birth. This insinuates that the parents-to-be are selfish, naive dreamers who would rather have a spiritual experience and in turn risk their baby's well-being. Frankly, I find this manipulative approach to be fear mongering, abhorrent, and that it is this very attitude that is the selfish and naive one to take.

First off, what is good for the mother—i.e., love, caring, trust, healthy relationships, etc.—translates into what is good for the baby, clinically speaking. Those immeasurable, real aspects of love and caring produce clinically measurable positive results for both mother and baby and, therefore, father, family, and society.

Take for example a study done by the Heart/Math Institute[16] that was conducted to determine if emotions have an effect on DNA. DNA typically has the form of a double helix—kind of looks like a winding staircase. The researchers took some DNA from a human placenta, which is pristine and has qualities that adult DNA no longer has. Twenty-eight vials of DNA were given (one each) to 28 trained researchers. Each researcher had been trained how to generate and *feel* feelings, and they each had strong emotions. They found that with directing positive emotions of gratitude, love, compassion, etc. to the DNA, the DNA began relax. The longer the focus of emotions went on, the intertwining strands of the DNA ultimately became no longer intertwined! The less intertwined our DNA strands are, the more our potential for growth is released and our immune system is strengthened. It also helps our cells divide and helps us to heal from injury more rapidly. Conversely, the study found that negative emotions such as rage, hate, and fear tighten up the twisting DNA and switch off many of its DNA codes. If you've ever felt "shut down" by negative emotions, now you know that your body was equally shut down.

In summary, if you love, trust, and nurture the mother, those emotions communicate and direct the infant's DNA to either be in a state of calm or agitation, which translates into states of health or illness, and in some cases life or death.[17]

Additionally, a number of studies[18] done on doulas showed that even though the doulas employed no clinical skills or intervention with tools, such as drugs, that their presence and the skills they bring to the labor room, which include calmness, love, patience and trust, produce a real measurable effect in the form of healthier outcomes for mothers and babies.

But let me go back to the statement "The most important thing is a healthy baby."

I've been sitting here for a while contemplating if this is actually the most true statement that could be made in the situation. In reality, I've contemplated it since the beginning of my journey on this birth road. I'm toying with the notion that maybe two other statements actually hold more truth.

Either, "The most important thing is that the baby *and* mother are healthy" or "The most important thing is that the mother is healthy"

Without you, the baby doesn't exist. Without you, the odds of the baby even surviving go down significantly. Yes, *you* are important. Say it, "I am important." Now say it out loud, with conviction, "I am important." You matter. Your health matters. Your mental state matters. Your emotional state matters. Your spiritual state matters. Your connection to your baby matters. The way you feel about yourself matters.

Let me tell you in detail why I've come to this conclusion.

In the old days, if a mother died during or shortly after childbirth, it was almost expected that the surviving infant would die, too. If the motherless baby wasn't essentially given to a wet nurse's family for at least the first year, there was little hope.

A U.S. woman's risk of dying in childbirth is today very low; although ranking No. 34 in the world is still unacceptably high in comparison to other developed nations.[19] It may be because a newborn and baby can be fed acceptable substitutes to breast milk to stay alive that we've marginalized and trivialized the importance of the mother's role in the survival of the infant, but does the mental and physical health of the postpartum mother have any effect on the viability of the baby? Of course!

Suppose that a modern-day mother died in childbirth, suddenly a whole host of survival questions come into play. This puts massive amounts of stress on the family and, in turn, the baby himself. This stress on the baby puts him at risk for failure to thrive, just to name one ailment of many.

But the most common scenario in the U.S. is that the mother is indeed alive, but physically, mentally, or spiritually isn't thriving. She's damaged, feeling incapable, like a failure, broken. This sounds like the perfect recipe for postpartum depression, doesn't it? How about personal neglect? Infant neglect? Breakdown of the marriage or relationships? Or maybe just years of recovery. This downward spiral puts the infant and family at literal risk.

The health of the mother *is* the health of the baby, the health of the mother *is* the health of the family; therefore, the health of the mother *is* the health of society, the nation, and the world.

It is vitally important that the birth goes well in favor of the mother, clinically speaking, psychologically speaking, and spiritually speaking. So is the most important thing that the baby is healthy? Think again. Your health is equally if not more important.

> *For the hand that rocks the cradle*
> *Is the hand that rules the world.*
> —*William Ross Wallace*

Yep, she rules, all right. For better or worse, it is our choice.

> *We are now discovering the long-term effect on families of treating women as if they were merely containers to be opened and relieved of their contents; and of concentrating on a bag of muscle and birth canal, rather than relating to and caring for the person to whom they belong.*
>
> —Sheila Kitzinger

Are there any limits to what you can achieve for your birth? Depending on who you talk to, the limits are everywhere and there are a lot of them. But are there really any limits?

Current scientific and physical limitations in birth are always changing; sometimes for better and sometimes for worse. What is standard and presented as truth today might be an archaic practice and mindset by the time your children are having babies.

I remember when my sister went into labor, and my mom reminded her that "She can't eat anything now that she's in labor." I knew full well why she was telling my sister that, but I played dumb and asked, "What do you mean?"

"Well, it's dangerous for her to eat food now," she said.

"Because her digestive system has stopped working?" I teased.

"No, she could die if she eats," my mom said.

"That's actually outdated information, Mom. If she doesn't keep hydrated and eat at least a little something, she won't have enough energy to push the baby out."

"Oh, well, that's what they always told me when I went into labor. I went 24 hours without food for you, Amy," she lamented.

This belief, NPO (no food by mouth), is actually still around today and promoted in some hospitals, even though there is absolutely no science to support it. It stems from the belief that every laboring woman is a presurgical patient and needs to be treated like one. The theory is that if a woman needed general anesthesia, having anything in her stomach would increase the risk of her vomiting and possibly aspirating the fluid into her lungs and possibly dying. Well, let me emphasize that this notion is a *theory*. The facts are:

> There is not a single documented case [in 20 years of medical history] of aspiration in an individual (not just pregnant women) who was properly anesthetized by today's standard of anesthesia whether the person has eaten or not.[20]

Goer also found that maternal death rate from aspiration with and without anesthesia is 2.6 deaths per *1 million*. That's less than .1 percent. And fasting (going without food or drink) actually *increases* your risk of aspiration should you have general anesthesia.[21]

In fact, in 2009 ACOG announced that it was relaxing its position on drinking in labor. No longer were women allowed only ice chips, but they stated it was now safe for women to have any clear fluid during labor and birth. Did women's biology somehow change in 2009 that all of the sudden it was safe to drink during labor? Of course not. It's always been safe to eat and drink during labor, it just took the ACOG decades to catch up with what women have always instinctively known.

My point is that science is fickle. Not to say it's not valid to consider, but only *consider* it. What is true today may be not true tomorrow, and in fact may be found to be a dangerous way to practice. Ultimately, you have to go with whatever beings you peace, whether the science agrees with it or not. I will tell you, though, that most people have an impossible time taking fear and risking social rejection out of decisions. Let me give you an extreme example to illustrate this point.

In my class, I ask people to answer the following question in their head:

"Are we going to circumcise if we have a girl?"

Of course, most people not only say out loud an annoyed, "No!", but also physically recoil at the thought because the question is so offensive to them. So, then I ask them to answer this next question in their head:

"Are we going to circumcise if we have a boy?"

The reactions are quite different. In fact, some people get offended at the thought of *not* circumcising a boy. Two opposite reactions to essentially the same question. Then I go on to ask them why they have a double standard. The first response usually is that there is no benefit and a lot of downsides to circumcising a girl.

"What if I told you there was benefit to female circumcision? What if I said I had multiple studies proving that a circumcised woman experiences and transmits fewer infections and diseases? Would that change your decision?"

I've never had a couple say yes. It just goes against what society believes, holds valuable, and is taught. But, with a boy, his genitalia are fair game. Our societal traditions are different. Why? Because studies prove this or that? Well, according to my little experiment in class, studies one way or the other have no bearing on decision making when it comes to circumcising your child. That can't be it, then. What is it? False tradition, fear of the unknown, social rejection and misinformation. But yet, if you ask someone why they chose circumcision, none of those factors come into play. Sometimes you happen to get someone who will honestly tell you, "So he doesn't look different. We wanted him and his dad to match." Are men in this country really so threatened by their little baby's penis? Are they really that insecure? I honestly would like to give men more credit than that. Would I feel threatened enough by my daughter's breasts that I would insist on plastic surgery so we look alike? No! That isn't it! It's just fear, plain and simple, but no one will recognize that. Fear of what? Well, the fears vary, but mostly it's fear of tribal or sexual rejection. Shoot, we imprison people in this country for removing a girl's foreskin, but insurance companies will even go so far as pay a doctor to take off a boy's foreskin.

So, my point is, really dig deep to pull out the fears that you think are fact. And who knows, they may be fact, but more likely than not, they are merely false traditions and misinformation that, for your sake and your baby's, need to be addressed today.

I could go on and on proving my points in regards to the changing tides and fads (yes, I said fads) of other birth practices such as episiotomy, Cesarean, VBAC, birth positions, pushing techniques, monitoring protocols, etc. Fads are ideas that catch on independent of whether or not they are scientifically verified or even make any sense. What is acceptable and touted as fact today was banned decades ago and vice versa. Most of what is practiced in the PABC is merely a fad, just like blood-letting, poodle skirts, MC Hammer pants, and the Atkins Diet. The birth practices and approaches that have been around for centuries are the real, time-tested practices that we should be giving heed to.

Here is a short list of outdated birth and parenting fads:
- Routine supine delivery—laying flat on your back to deliver.
- Twilight sleep—knocking a woman completely out to deliver, only to have her wake up days later.
- DES (diethylstilbestrol)—used in the '50s and '60s to prevent miscarriage, but it also severely deformed babies.
- Thalidomide—used in the late '50s to curb morning sickness with grave effects on offspring.
- Restricted weight gain—for quite a while many women were only allowed to gain 15–20 pounds and were prescribed diuretics to keep their weight down.
- Routine episiotomy—as in *everyone* got an episiotomy.
- Routine forceps—as in *everyone* had forceps used on them.
- Banning fathers from the delivery room
- Routine restraints in labor and birth—as in *all* women had their wrists and ankles tied to the bed.
- Sterile draping—the blue paper that they drape over women's bottom half during the pushing stage.
- NPO—no food or water by mouth.
- Routine repeat Cesareans—which was the standard for about 20 years, then women fought to make VBAC a viable option in the hospital, and currently it is now a fad again. It is increasingly difficult to have access to a hospital VBAC.
- Routine bottle feeding and/or sugar water supplementation until mother's milk comes in.
- Routine infant/mother separation
- Routine circumcision

Short list of modern-day birth and parenting fads:
- Routine IV
- Epidurals

- Elective induction
- Elective Cesarean
- Internal fetal monitoring
- Continuous external fetal monitoring
- Ultrasound (intravaginal and external)
- Banning hospital waterbirth
- Routine hospitalization
- Routine repeat Cesareans
- Routine Cesarean for breech presentation
- Male circumcision
- Solitary infant sleep—putting infants to sleep in a separate room from the mother.
- Infant "crying it out"—the practice and theory that letting babies, even newborns, cry themselves to sleep will ease bedtime and make for a more independent child.
- Scheduled breast feeding
- Routine use of a pacifier
- Carrying your baby around in a car seat

I recognize and validate that every mother/baby pair is different and may come with their own unique set of concerns, but I'm merely proposing that what you espouse as fact or beneficial, your hard-and-fast excuses, should be re-examined. In all likelihood you have choices; in fact, many of them. Your peaceful birth may be more within your reach than you think. Right now, you may not know exactly how you will achieve it, but something inside of you is telling you that there is another, better way. If you honor that small voice of peace, you will always be led in the right direction and make the best choices.

> I find it fascinating that most people plan their vacations with better care than they plan their lives. Perhaps it's because escape is easier than change.
> —Jim Rohn, motivational speaker

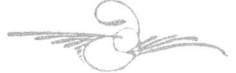

# What Is Possible

I've been a birth doula and independent childbirth educator since 1997. I've become close friends with birth professionals who have been in the field for much longer than I. I've known secondhand, and have also witnessed with my own eyes and heart, many miracles.

## The Dionnes' Birth

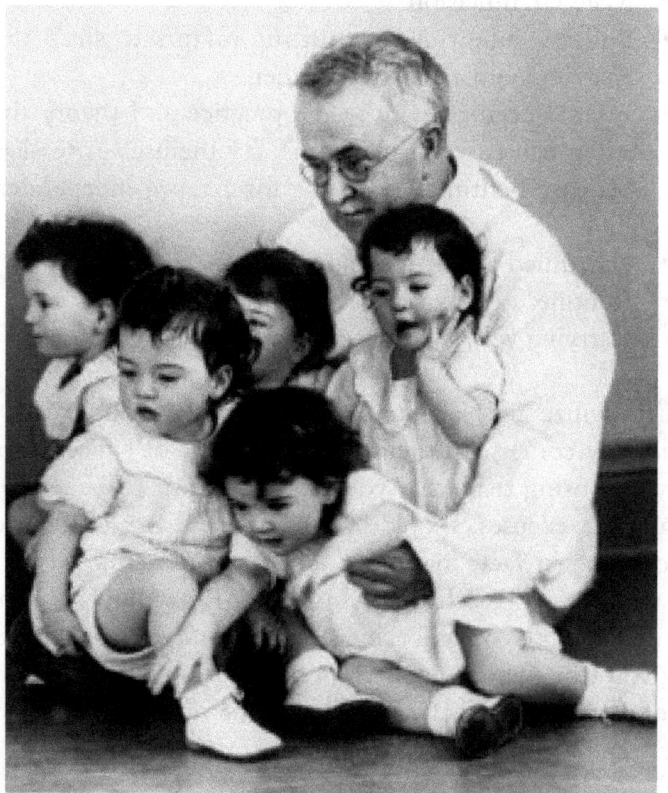

This is a short retelling of the Dionne quintuplets, born in 1934. This was before fertility drugs, ultrasounds, incubators, mass hospitalizations, and sadly it was the beginning of devaluing human breast milk, which makes the quintuplets' story even more miraculous.

The Dionnes were a farming family with five previous children named Ernest, Rose Marie, Therese, Daniel, and Pauline, who was only eleven months older than the quints.

The Dionnes also had three sons after the quintuplets. Oliva Jr., Victor, and Claude (the last son was born when the quintuplets were 12.)

Elzire, the mother, suspected she was carrying twins, but no one was aware that quintuplets were even possible. The quintuplets were born two months premature. Later genetic tests showed that the girls were identical and were created from one single egg cell. Elzire reported having had cramps in her third month and passing a strange object, which may have been a sixth fetus.

Dr. Allan Roy Dafoe is credited with assisting at the birth of the quintuplets. Originally, he diagnosed Elzire with a "fetal abnormality." He assisted at the home birth with the help of two midwives, Aunt Donalda and Madam Benoit Lebel, who were summoned by Oliva Dionne in the middle of the night.

Their birth order, weight and measurement were not recorded; all that is known is that the three bigger ones were born first. The quintuplets were immediately wrapped in cotton sheets and old napkins and laid in the corner of the bed. Dr. Dafoe was certain none of the babies could live. Shortly after the births were completed, Elzire went into shock and Dafoe thought she would die as well, but she recovered in two hours.

The babies were kept in an ordinary wicker basket borrowed from the neighbors, with heated blankets. They were brought into the kitchen and set by the open door of the stove to keep warm. One by one, they were taken out of the basket and massaged with olive oil. Every two hours, for the first twenty-four, they were fed water sweetened with corn syrup. By the second day they were moved to a slightly larger laundry basket, and kept warm with hot-water bottles. They were watched constantly and often had to be roused. They were then fed with "seven-twenty" formula; that is, cow's milk, boiled water, two spoonfuls of corn syrup, and one or two drops of rum for a stimulant.[22]

## Mozambique Miracle Baby

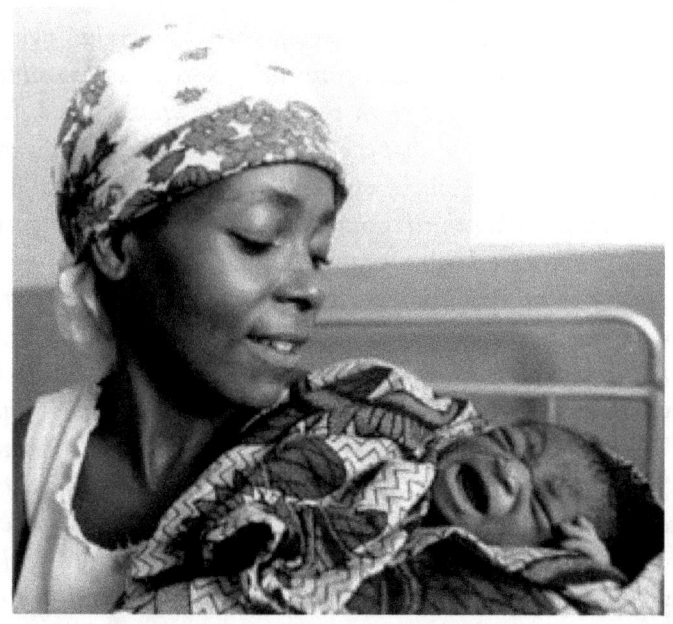

It was a miracle amid the misery of Mozambique's floods. Above the rising waters, heavily pregnant Sophia Pedro clung to life for three days before giving birth on a tree branch as the filthy flood torrents swirled below. The brave mother and her newborn were then plucked to safety by a helicopter crew in a scene captured by a television cameraman and beamed around the world.

It transformed Sophia, who has no formal education and has spent her life hoeing vegetables on a tiny farmstead, into an international icon of courage and motherhood. Newly reunited with her husband Salvador, who only learnt of his wife's ordeal weeks later, Sophia revealed her fears and helplessness at the pain of the contractions, her struggle through the process of giving birth and her awe at experiencing a human miracle which moved millions around the world.

The drama began when Sophia carried her children Benito, [aged] two, and her four-year-old daughter, Celina, to the branches of a nearby mafura tree, similar to an Irish ash, to escape the overflowing Limpopo river that swept away their home and possessions in a remote area of the country. Speaking through an interpreter Sophia, 23, with baby Rositha in her arms, told the Irish Examiner:

"When the flood came all I could think of was saving my children. I picked up Benito and strapped him to my back, as I do when I'm working in the fields. My daughter I just carried in my arms, holding her above the water swirling around my chest.

"We were all so frightened. Surely we were going to die. We had seen the bodies of our neighbors in the water. I prayed to God to save us and yet it would be impossible for me to swim. With no time for any discussion, all of us clung to the lower branches of the three big trees nearby and scrambled as high as we could.

"We somehow found branches to rest in and stayed there, waiting for help. As night fell, I became terrified for my children's lives and for my baby. We were all so hungry. There was nothing for us to eat and nothing to drink but drops of rain. It was humid and steamy and all the while the floods were getting higher and higher.

"Salvador's mother never left my side as we tried to comfort the children by singing and praying. If we slept we would fall, maybe drown, so the family. worked to keep each other awake."

After the first 24 hours, Salvador's grandmother, in her 70s, slipped into the water and was washed away as the others looked helplessly on.

"We prayed for her soul and for each other," Sophia continued. "We are Christians and we sang every hymn we knew." As dawn broke on the third day, Sophia felt the familiar pain of contractions.

"I knew the baby was coming and I was terrified. I knew we could not get to a hospital and there was no way we could get help. I did not know what would happen. Salvador's mother comforted me and the children.

"I had given up hope and then, unbelievably, come the sound of a helicopter. Out of the heavens had come help. I felt confusion because I didn't know what was happening, I thought they had come to rescue all of us but they only wanted to take the children. I didn't speak their language and couldn't tell them I was about to give birth."

They flew away with my children and my relief turned to despair. There I was, still on the tree, about to give birth. I consoled myself that at least my son and daughter would survive this.

"The birth was over quite quickly. It is a painful experience anyway and in the tree it was dreadful. There was blood everywhere; a terrible mess. But nothing can take away from the joy of seeing a new life enter the world."

Salvador's mother, also named Rositha, recalls the moment equally vividly.

"I held her, with nothing to wrap her in but the clothes I was wearing, all of us covered in perspiration, rain and blood."

Emergency crews from the world's aid agencies were giving priority to children but, as the South African helicopter winched a man down to save Benito and Celina, he had realised the young mother was in labour and needed urgent help.

The helicopter took the children to relief workers half an hour away and collected a male nurse, who was flown to the scene and lowered into the tree just in time to cut the newborn's umbilical cord. A few minutes later Sophia and baby were winched away to safety. The TV cameraman captured the scene despite the fear of his own helicopter causing a down-draught which threatened the stability of the trees.

"I knew I was witnessing a moment of humanity that I might never see again," he says now.

Sophia and her baby were briefly treated in hospital. Rositha was weighed at about 5lb. They then joined the other family survivors at the Wenela refugee camp in Chibuto.

—BBC, 2000

We do not know the full range of our own possibilities. After all, only a few decades ago you would have been laughed at if you would have told someone that you'd be able to send a letter around the world in a matter of seconds, and for free no less. It is vital for you to embrace and accept that miracles happen in birth all the time, every day. No matter what you've been told, experienced, or think you know, what you think is impossible can truly be possible.

You have not yet given birth to this child. The path for your baby's delivery is not set in stone. You can create something different, something better than what you have planned right now.

Where do you want to have your baby? I'm going to ask you again, and this time drop your excuses and fears. If you could have your ideal birth, where would you want it to be? A surgery room? A hospital room? A birth center? A home? Outdoors?

How long do you want your birth to be? Who do you want with you? Have you let yourself even explore that? Why not? The possibilities are endless. Don't be afraid to ask, explore, and dream.

> So many of our dreams at first seem impossible, then they seem improbable, and then, when we summon the will, they soon become inevitable.
> —Christopher Reeve

# 3

# Taking Responsibility, Owning Your Power, Claiming Your Birthright

*Anything I've ever done that ultimately was worthwhile . . . initially scared me to death.*

—Betty Bender

The first family dentist I chose, I kind of settled for. There wasn't really anyone in my area that practiced the kind of dentistry I was looking for, so I picked an acquaintance who I thought was "good enough." When I rejected fluoride treatments, I got a lecture. When I insisted on composite fillings rather than amalgam for my kids' baby teeth, I got a lecture *and* got laughed at. When I rejected general anesthesia and insisted on a local for work on my kids, I got an eye roll and another lecture. Sheesh, how many lectures did I need? Can't I take a hint? Leave, Amy! Find a new dentist! It's not like there's a shortage of them. Go, woman, go! But I didn't.

After one visit, where I had let myself be talked into a metal cap put on my daughter's baby molar, as we were buckling our seat belts to go home, I asked my then 6-year-old daughter how the visit went (since I wasn't "allowed" back with her. What a mistake).

"It was good, I guess."

"What did they do?"

"I sat down in the chair and they put this thing over my mouth and nose and told me to breathe in."

*This is odd,* I thought.

"And then what?" I probed.

"I don't know. It was weird, I went to sleep."

*Uh . . . WHAT?!*

Holy schamoley, I was fuming inside. They didn't ask, I didn't consent. How could they give my baby general anesthesia without asking?

I have this thing about anesthesia. I'm not the biggest of fans. I'm especially not the biggest of fans using it willy-nilly and on my kids. I am *very* careful about it. Just the month before, my friend had told me about her dentist, who had put his 7-year-old under general, and well, let's just say the kid didn't wake up. Horrifying! So, I'm just coming off of digesting this story and feeling so sympathetic for this poor family, when this happens.

Maybe I should have waited. No, I *know* I should have waited, but when I got home, I raced to my bedroom, picked up the phone, shut the door so I wasn't interrupted (or maybe it was so my kids couldn't hear), and immediately called the dentist's office.

"So, my daughter tells me that she slept through her appointment." I'm trying to stay calm, but there's a tone in my voice, with an edge to it, and an eagerness to pounce.

"Uh, okaaaayyyy," the poor receptionist says nervously.

"I don't understand. How did she sleep through getting a cap on? Can you explain that?" I'm still trying to stay calm. I realized it wasn't this poor receptionist's fault or doing, but she was the one who picked up the phone.

"Well, let me give you to the dental assistant who helped."

*Yeah, I don't blame you. I can't even imagine the hurried, hushed conversation that happened between her and the assistant in that 30 seconds. Hand it over, sister, quickly.*

"Hi, Mrs. Jones? I hear you have some questions about your daughter's visit?"

"I'm wondering how she slept through getting a cap on." I said, trying to stay calm.

"Well, we gave her some anesthesia," she said slowly and in a high-pitched, lullaby, sing-song voice—which bothers me a lot.

"What kind?" I said back, mimicking her tone. I know, I know, I'm working on not doing that. It's horribly rude.

She cleared her throat, "General," she said tentatively.

"Is there protocol on getting parental consent before administering general anesthesia?" There was a hint of annoyance in my voice.

"Well, it's just so common that most parents don't mind if—"

I cut her off, "I don't know if you've noticed, but I'm not most parents. Most parents let their kids eat deep fried Ding Dongs everyday and run around with Pixy Stix in their mouth. Have you ever seen my kids with Pixy Stix or Ding Dongs?"

"No, but, um, well we didn't think—"

I cut her off again, "Obviously." I *know*! I shouldn't be mean like that. I'm working on it, okay?

"Has she had complications?" the assistant desperately trying to get me to focus on "what's most important."

"What if I told you she has?" I let a few seconds go by to give her time to digest what it meant if she had had complications. "Look, by *laaaaaww*, aren't you supposed to get my consent for general?" I drew out the word *law* make her realize that she has a possible lawsuit on her hands.

"Well, I'm not sure, it's never been an issue before," she said sheepishly.

"That's 'cause you have idiot patients. It's an issue now."

There was an uncomfortable pause as she was trying to find the words to diffuse this situation.

"I'm so sorry, Mrs. Jones. In the future—"

I cut her off again, "In the future you won't need my consent because we won't be there to give it."

"Wait, Mrs. Jones—" Click.

Oh, I was mad, that was for sure. And that well-deserved tongue lashing I gave her, that made me feel all better, right? No. I was mad at them for days. And when I got done being mad at them, I got mad at myself.

I knew better. I really wasn't an idiot. So, why on earth did I act like one? I did something unusual in this society. I took responsibility. I stepped back, and stopped blaming them for my bad choices. Yes, of course they should have gotten my consent. I bet they get it from parents now. But ultimately this situation was *my* fault. Here is where I screwed up, in chronological order for your reading pleasure:

1. I didn't know exactly what I wanted from a dentist. I had an idea, but that's not good enough.
2. I didn't try hard enough. Even if I couldn't find one who fit even close to my ideal, I could have at least found one who was respectful and prioritized seeking full, informed consent. Come to find out only a few years later, there were two great dentists that surpassed my ideal only two hours north of me! It would have been a drive, but, in hindsight, well worth it to have a caregiver whose philosophies matched mine.
3. I certainly didn't do my due diligence. Did I even really interview any dentists? No. Did I even ask my like-minded friends their feedback on their dentists? No. I only called maybe five dentists and interviewed none of them. I just gave up after the fifth because none of them even remotely resembled what I thought I wanted. Let's just say that last year, I interviewed eight, yes eight, orthodontists and researched my options like crazy. I would have done more, but No. 8 was my orthodontist prince charming.
4. I didn't communicate well enough. I should have put in writing, in my files, the terms of our relationship. What was acceptable, unacceptable, and possibly negotiable to me. This would have required some minor footwork and research on my part, but instead I just put my hands over my ears, pursed my lips and shut my eyes and crossed my fingers. Yes, I thought those little lectures were me speaking up enough, but now I realized they just put me in the category of paranoid mom and dismissed every position and concern I had.

For some reason, I thought I was going to change a lion into a lamb. Had I implemented those four steps and been proactive, I likely wouldn't have had that experience, or even hired him, for that matter. Come to think of it, why wasn't he the one on the phone with me? The point is I deceived myself into thinking that I could ultimately get what I wanted if I stood my ground firmly and nicely enough. I should have just written them a nice letter letting them know why I was leaving and had that be it. As my good friend, Jonelle, puts it:

> *Hiring a caregiver or choosing a birthplace that's not in line with your philosophies and priorities and then insisting they change the way they do things to accommodate you is like walking into Walmart and demanding they carry one particular line of organic products just for you, and by the way . . . you want those organic products now.*

While it'd be great if your caregiver and birthplace turned their protocols on their heads just for you, the truth is that permanent change takes time and collective demand from the majority of women. If you don't agree with your caregiver's or birthplace's policies and philosophies, *hire someone else.* I'm giving you permission right here, that you can leave. Women do it every day.

If you don't switch caregivers and/or birthplace, and your birth doesn't go the way you like because of the care they gave you, who is it that you should blame? Them? Or yourself? If you are now listing all the reasons why you are stuck with your chosen caregiver and birthplace, stop. I'm serious, stop right now. You are not the first woman who has had this barrier in your path. You are not a victim. You have choices. I've seen women from all walks of life—rich, poor, short, tall, thin, not so thin (you are pregnant, after all)—go to extreme lengths to achieve what they've felt is right for their births.

Money, proximity, family circumstances, health conditions, convenience, it's all workable and, for the most part, just your perception. What seems huge and monumental to you, is really no big deal to someone else who is in your same shoes. Choose to see it as a bump in the road, not a mountain to climb, and it will be easy, or at least easier. This is *your* birth, *you're* the one who has to live with the outcome, *you're* the one making the decisions, *you're* in charge. You don't need to fight. In fact, the destructive energy of fighting will work against you. Just start doing, moving forward in the direction you want to go. You don't need anyone's permission or approval. Like the adage says, where there's a will, there's a way.

By the way, I got my karma back today. I was pulling into the store parking lot and saw a man and his little boy out of the corner of my eye to my right, but in my view, they weren't yet crossing the street. So, I didn't slow down or anything. After I pulled in a parking space and got done giving my kids instructions on getting out of the car and into the store safely, as I pulled on the car handle to open the door, I looked up, and here is this man and his son standing there.

"Hi, how are you?" I said a little confused.

"Did you see us standing in that crosswalk?" he asked calmly.

"I saw you standing there but it didn't look to me like you were crossing." I said.

"Well, we were at the crosswalk ready to walk, and you didn't slow down a bit," he said a little more defensively.

At this point, I'm thinking he just wants an apology, so I said, "I am sorry, sir. I truly thought you weren't crossing."

"My son is only 3 and a half. Do you know how impulsive three-and-a-half-year-olds are?" I could tell he's gearing up for a fight.

"Sir, I have five children. I know how it is, I understand. I am sorry." I repeated.

"I just can't believe that—"

I shouldn't have, but I cut him off. I had just gotten done with an hour-long natural family planning consultation that I had to take my kids with me to because I lost my babysitter last minute.

"Sir, I am sorry, I understand what you are saying. I really don't think I need a lecture."

He then started going into gory detail about his job, which was handling accidents. Well, then I knew all he wanted to do was be right and tell me off, so I shut my car door and "politely" drove away. In hindsight, I should have asked him what he wanted me to do or say to make him happy, but I was tired and annoyed. As I drove away, immediately I knew it was my karma for giving the dental assistant an earful and never apologizing. It never does anyone any good to tell them off. Note to self: Apologize when you need to apologize!

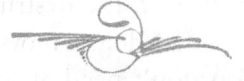

# Why Do You Want a Peaceful Birth?

At first blush, this may seem like a silly question. Who, after all, wants a dramatic or tragic birth? Well, let's think about that. I'm serious, Who do you know who subconsciously would want a dramatic birth? I can almost guarantee you that you know someone, on some level, who would love the attention and power that having a dramatic birth would bring. Maybe that someone is even you.

Have you ever seen that *Saturday Night Live* skit with Penelope? She's always wanting to one-up whoever's talking, every time taking it to unbelievable extremes.

> Nicole: *It's nice to meet you. So, how do you know Sue and Anthony?*
>
> Penelope: *We're really good friends. So—we've known each other for a really long time. I just know them really well. Probably better than a lot of people here, so—*
>
> Glenn: *Oh—oh, well, uh—we met them at Lamaze class, six months ago.*
>
> Penelope: *I've known them for, like, seven years. So, just a little bit longer. I've just known them for a really long time, so—longer, just better friends. So—longer than you guys. So—*
>
> Sue: *Hey! Attention! Attention, everyone! Um—can I have everyone's attention? Uh—first of all, I just want to say thank you—*
>
> Penelope: *I also want to thank everybody for coming.*
>
> Sue: *Um—on behalf of Anthony and I, I just wanted to thank all of you for coming tonight—*
>
> Penelope: *Thank all of you for coming tonight.*
>
> Sue: *We-we feel so blessed—*
>
> Penelope: *I feel really blessed, too—a lot of really good things in my life, you know?*
>
> Sue: *Not only for this new home—*
>
> Penelope: *I have a new house, too—it's really big.*
>
> Sue: *But for all of our amazing friends—*
>
> Penelope: *I have a lot of friends, too—a lot of friends—*
>
> Glenn: *She really doesn't stop, does she? Hey, Penelope? Guess what. I have a cousin that lives in space, and I recently lost five hundred pounds, and you know what? My wife and I got here by paddling a kayak down the street, and two minutes after my baby was born, she spoke French.*

> Penelope: *That's—all I have to say is: I have sixty cousins that live in space and other dimensions, um—I just lost seven hundred pounds, and, um, I invented kayaks, and I invented the streets, so—um—I have six babies now, who spoke forty-four languages before they came out of my stomach, um—and, uh—I can fly, so—*[23]

This is just an extreme example of what happens in most female social circles, and it's important to note and admit to yourself if you do it. Have you ever noticed that conversations with groups of women very easily gravitate toward the topic of birth? I used to think it was because I was in the conversations, that somehow I was steering the talk that direction because I love birth so much. It used to drive me crazy because inevitably the women would start telling one horror story after another, one defeat after another, one self-deprecating remark after another.

I was sick of this. So, I started removing myself from most female-only conversations and started just eavesdropping. I'd pretend I was grazing at the buffet table, or programming my cell phone, or just close my eyes and appear to be resting. And what did I find out? It wasn't me influencing the conversation! I realized that when mothers get together, they talk about a lot of things, but one of the most common of topics are pregnancy, birth, breast-feeding, postpartum, and parenting. Which would be fantastic if it weren't such an enormous drag to listen to.

Mom's groups, church, work, parties, you name it, they'll talk about birth. And baby showers are the worst. THE WORST!

It's almost a competition between them to trump the other's experience. Baby showers are where I can feel most alone, because I've got nothing but good to say about my own pregnancy and birth experiences and all the births I've attended. And when someone has nothing but positive to say, competition to be "on top" disappears. There is no contest in who had the most loving, peaceful experience.

The majority, about 90+ percent of American women, are on this level in my opinion. They have pain, grief, bitterness, resentment, and negativity about their birth experiences, as do mass media. I remember back in 2002 that our mom's group wanted to put out a news segment about the viability of doing a VBAC in the current non-VBAC-friendly climate where we lived. It was met with a lot of hostility by the news producer in charge of those types of segments because she herself was talked into having repeated Cesareans. We were booed right out of there because of the bias in the local newsroom. That tribal mentality is pervasive, convincing, and viral.

Most parents-to-be know what they don't want:

- They don't want a Cesarean.
- They don't want forceps or vacuum extraction.
- They don't want a difficult birth.
- They don't want hostility.

Which is a great start, but for most, that's where their wish list ends.

The way that our tribal birth mentality leads us in our conversation and media gives us a great idea of what we don't want. But it feels so good to gripe, whine, pass on responsibility, and grieve. We feel validated and in good company. For those few moments that you are recounting your heroics, the weight of your dramatic birth is lifted. In a way, it can seem almost healing for those few moments.

But what this part of our PABC does is keep us in fear, doubt, pain, and submission. Any good midwife will tell you that as a training midwife, you will attract the very births you are afraid to attend. In the same vein, women can attract the births they are terrified of, because they are so focused on the thing they want to avoid.

I always take a deep breath when a woman or couple says they've made a decision based on a fear of what they don't want.

"We're having a home birth because we're afraid of the hospital."

I make a mental note that if that fear isn't replaced with faith and they don't accept the hospital as a viable option, then their odds of a successful home birth just reduced.

"I'm planning a natural birth because I have a fear of needles."

Again, I'm make a mental note that the likelihood that needles will become part of her birth experience just increased.

"I'm having a planned C-section because I'm afraid of all the unknowns in vaginal birth."

I then say a quick prayer that she doesn't encounter the myriad of unknowns that can come with a Cesarean.

Even if your decision is ultimately the right one for you, I've learned that the reasons *why* you choose something—in other words, the spirit of your decision—matters immensely. It impacts not only the clinical outcome of the birth, but also the psychological and spiritual outcome.

When you're putting your energy on avoiding a Cesarean, you are still focusing on a Cesarean! Why not put your energy to better, more productive use and focus on a vaginal birth? When you focus your energy on avoiding needles, your thoughts are still being drawn to the needles. Instead, focus on the organic movements of a normal birth.

If you want a peaceful, healthy, loving birth, you *have* to put your energy there. Focusing on what you don't want will increase the odds that whatever you are focusing on will more likely come to fruition.

By grasping the fact that this tribal mentality is what most women chose to join in on, you can make a conscious choice to join another tribe. Yes, there *is* another tribe. And it's a whole lot more fun, happy, and sane than the predominant one. But, alas, as of today it's still a small one to join. But it's been growing incrementally for decades.

This tribe talks about the joys of pregnancy, birth, breast-feeding, and parenting. This tribe is unified in their resolve and commitment to peaceful birth. This tribe is faithful to the fact that birth works and is amazing. Is this tribe perfect? Well, I have to admit that its members have their fair share of bumps in the road. But with the collective knowledge, love, and positive energy this tribe generates, problems get solved quickly and relatively smoothly. It's awesome and functions at a higher and healthier level than the PABC tribe, no doubt.

This tribe chooses to see and manifest the peaceful births and miracles you are seeking. Every so often, a rogue member of the PABC tribe accidentally gets a peak into the other tribe and will get a whiff of what things could be like. Most of the time they bury what they learned from the other tribe in the sand and go on making up or exaggerating something dramatic from their birth-year experience when they are in their PABC circles. If they don't, then they become outsiders, and an outsider sparks discussion. Those in the

PABC tribe would have to re-examine their birth philosophies and experiences and may end up changing. Change, after all, isn't exactly on the PABC's agenda. Stick to the status quo, do it like the rest of them, and you'll belong. Don't be the tall poppy.

> Just as a woman's heart knows how and when to pump, her lungs to inhale, and her hand to pull back from fire, so she knows when and how to give birth.
>
> —Virginia di Orio

### Same Woman, Two Natural Childbirths, Two Different Outcomes

*My first two births were typical, medicated, and managed births. I was happy with them, so when I had my son, Nicholas, I was prepared to check into the hospital, get an epidural, and have them wake me up when it was time to push. I had no intention or training to have him naturally. So when I did check into the hospital too late for that epidural, it was panic time.*

*I remember grabbing (well, clawing, really) the nurse's arm and demanding that she give me a crash course on that "breathing thing" that I knew women did to get through the monstrous pain. But the time for Lamaze training had come and gone, and I clung on the verge of completely losing it. My mom reports that I woke her up in the waiting room with my screaming. I remember staring at the clock, thinking that I could survive five more minutes, but after that I would die. I wanted to die. I wanted anything but to be having a nine-pound baby naturally.*

*When the baby's head crowned is when I really lost it. From that point on I just screamed, with my eyes squeezed shut and rendering permanent nail marks in my husband's arm. I was still screaming, when I heard somewhere out of oblivion my doctor calmly asserting,*

"Tyla, open your eyes. Open your eyes, Tyla." Without missing a beat in my continuous cries of terror, I squinted my eyes open just enough, to see her standing there holding my son. He had come out and I hadn't even noticed. In my head I was still birthing him, even though he was out already. Did I want to hold him? Let's just say I needed a few minutes to myself first. I felt like I had passed through death for him, but was it a beautiful experience? Not a bit.

Because of this experience, I did not want to be caught off-guard again. I really did feel a special bond with Nicholas (when I finally got around to holding him), and I just physically felt better after his natural birth than I had after my medicated births. I loved how alert and bright he seemed right after the birth, and my recovery was a cinch. So I was determined to be prepared for the birth of my daughter, two years later. I hired a doula, learned that "breathing thing," made up a birth plan, bought a whole lot of essential oils, and emotionally and mentally prepared myself to have her without any medication.

My daughter's birth was one of the most beautiful experiences of my entire life. I felt connected to all women who had ever lived, and a spiritual connection that I had never before experienced. It was still painful delivering all 10 pounds of her, but I knew what to expect this time, I had help beside me, and I had done the emotional and mental work to prepare for it. I was still laughing between contractions when I was dilated to a 9 with Clara, a far cry from the nurse-abuse that was happening at that point with the delivery of my son!

—Tyla, mother of four

> Rain, after all, is only rain; it is not bad weather. So also, pain is only pain; unless we resist it, then it becomes torment.
>
> —The I Ching

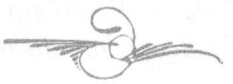

## Raising the (Birth) Bar

About a year after I began teaching childbirth education classes, I began to notice something. On the first night of the series, most of the moms-to-be would come with eagerness and excitement, and most of the men showed up with apprehension and a bit of confusion. It was the "I don't know why I'm here, my lady just told me I had to be here" look. Even though I try to be as clear and concise as possible in my literature, I fully understand the dads' position. After all, my husband came into the first of our own childbirth education classes with the same look.

Poor guys. Who knows what they think they are getting themselves into. Is it that they are afraid they'll have to look at pictures they don't want to look at? Do they think they are going to have to rehearse a bunch of "hee hee who who" breathing techniques? Or get themselves in odd, vulnerable positions?

Even though I do my best to put them at ease and joke around and be down to earth on the first night of class. I am the authority figure in their eyes, and that evokes some insecurity.

Inevitably throughout the class series, the couples forge friendships and find out that others in the class share their priorities, views, and philosophies. They find a new tribe. That, in and of itself, serves as a major stepping-stone to their peaceful birth. In fact, many of my former students from my first few years of teaching are still good friends to this day, 10+ years after their births.

But my absolute favorite part of teaching my childbirth education classes is the last night of class or the reunion class. These same people who walked through my doors for the first time like a deer in headlights have transformed into confident, knowledgeable, centered, stronger people. They leave my class knowing that *they* are the ultimate authority on their body, birth, and baby. Not me, not their midwife, OB, or nurse.

Now, of course, not all of the women and couples leave my classes taking on this new transformed self. But most of them do, and they affect others around them, which ultimately affects the local birth community, which impacts the national and global birth culture.

Because people left my childbirth class feeling so empowered and having the peaceful births they dreamed of, word spread like a new religion about my series and I got to the point where I had to refer people to other childbirth educators. People from all walks of life, who were from all over the world came to my classes. A stuntwoman, a policeman, a fireman, a lawyer, an acrobat, a nurse, a fertility doctor, a teacher, a professional singer, a model, an accountant, Polish, French, Canadian, Swiss, Mexican, you name it. This transformation truly transcended all boundaries. But, why wouldn't it? What people want out of their birth experience—a peaceful birth—is, by and large, universal. And peaceful birth resonates with just about everyone everywhere.

Deep down, people want to elevate themselves, be at peace, and heal. And I prayed fervently before each class I taught that I would be led in the right ways to inspire them to accomplish just that.

You might be saying, "But I don't have that in my area." Well, there are no excuses these days. First of all, start asking around, search the Internet for local groups. If none exist, you have two choices. Either create a group or settle for joining an online group, either one close to you or a national one. There are multiple places you can find support, education, and motivation. There really are no excuses. You can find the education and support you need, it may just take some digging.

In order to do this, though, you are likely going to have to go out of your comfort zone. Obviously, you can't learn new information and gain adequate support and clinical care by just turning to your neighbor and friends like in the old days. If you could, you wouldn't even be reading this book. You would already be far down the road to your peaceful birth. You will have to seek out additional friends, new caregivers, new environments, and new paradigms.

So, take a step back and take inventory. Think about where you want your birth to go and accept that you might need help from people outside your current tribe.

I am well aware that, for most of you reading this book, your greatest barrier (besides yourself) to achieving a peaceful birth is someone, or multiple people, in your tribe.

So, who is it? Your mother? Mother-in-law? Father? Best friend? Sister? Sister-in-law? Your husband? I've been doing this long enough to know just how much of an influence their fear for you and your unborn baby can be. But, I am going to say the following in an unequivocal term. It is *their* fear. Let it be their fear, not yours. The likelihood of you inspiring them to replace their fears with faith in the short amount of time before you have before you deliver your baby is slim. You cannot control them or force them to believe anything. Their greatest teacher will be your peaceful and confident example.

But can you reject their beliefs and their fears without rejecting them personally? Of course! Can you still achieve your peaceful birth without their support? Of course! It may require a shift in your relationship with them, which can seem scary. And your decisions, if they have been made known to them, can result in some pretty harsh treatment of you. But never once have I seen such a situation end in divorce or dismemberment from their tribe.

Of course there are some relationships that can be temporarily set aside for the sake of achieving your goals—acquaintances, co-workers, caregivers, etc. But if your family isn't destructive or abusive, they shouldn't be, nor do they need to be, set aside.

So, how do you hug a porcupine? I totally understand the instinctual desire to have the literal and emotional support and connection with your mother, sister, husband, and family during such a pivotal and critical time in your life. Ideally, you *should* have their support. You *deserve* their support. You were *meant* to have their support.

But just because you should have their support and you deserve it, doesn't mean you're going to get it. It's a gift they have to choose to give to you and sadly many pregnant and birthing women are denied this gift because their decisions run counter to their tribe's status quo for birth. *You* are the one who is intimately and literally connected to this child. You, first and foremost, have your baby's interest at heart, and you are the expert on how to bring this child into the world safely *and* peacefully. Your baby's blood is your blood, his cells are your cells, your emotions are his emotions. The mother-unborn-baby connection is on a whole different and unique level, one rarely recognized by science and certainly not understood by someone who has chosen to never emotionally connect with the child growing inside of them. The sooner you accept the possibility that you may not get the support from your closest loved ones that you desire, and you surrender to it, let go of your "need" for it, and come to a place of being happy without it, the more likely you are to get it.

Hopefully the following story will help comfort you, give you strength, and guide you to the bigger picture.

> I was highly educated, well read, and had an established career under way when I conceived our first child. But apparently, I was also naive and arrogant. I thought that just because I was educated and felt right about having my baby at home, my family would back me up. No such luck. I gleefully announced at a family function that we had decided to have a home birth. My family, being well acquainted with not holding back, gave me squinty-eyed stares that turned into a collective, "What are you thinking?" I was in my second trimester when I made this announcement and what culminated from there was heartbreaking.
>
> At first, I experienced belittlement, especially from my parents. I've never had a baby, how could I know the dangers or pain, they asked. I don't know what I'm getting myself into, they informed me. Had I ever seen a baby or mother die? Yes, these were the fearful words coming at me. Then it turned into flat-out rejection. They would never forgive me if my baby died. How could I do this to them? It's selfish. I was emailed and sent, almost daily, articles of horrific birth outcomes. Quickly I learned to just trash them outright and ignore them. It had gotten to the point where they tried to avoid me and wouldn't talk to me. They even tried to intimidate my midwife and doula away from attending me. We were a close family, or so I thought, and the anger and isolation from them created a pain I had neither anticipated nor thought I'd ever experience.
>
> A few weeks before my due date, small attempts were made by everyone to repair the damage that had been done. They realized I wasn't changing my mind and they had choices to make. I am grateful they chose to mend fences. After I had my baby beautifully at home, the waters were still a bit choppy, and I grieved the lack of support and ohhing and ahhing that I had so longed for from my

*parents. We had always had such a close relationship, and they let this one decision of mine bring them to the brink of destruction. It wasn't until I had my fourth child at home that they finally came around to accepting and integrating this decision of mine into their lives. In hindsight, I wish I would have only kept my decision to myself for the sake of a sane pregnancy; but I also wouldn't have approached it so naively. I made my fair share of mistakes in handling their reaction, which didn't help things. As much as I wanted a supportive, loving family connection during my pregnancies and births, that wasn't anything I could control. If I had just been more prepared for that, a lot of wasted time and hurt feelings could have been avoided.*

—Maggie, mother of four

To put it a little more bluntly, those loved ones around you may very well stand in the way of your having the birth you want. They will either be ignorant and fearful or grieving their own experiences and therefore will try to discourage you from moving forward. Or they will want the best for you and help you accomplish your goals. The latter are the only ones you should consider consulting and seeking assistance from. The first group, love them and keep them on a need-to-know basis.

Every once in a while I'll have clients or students that have hired me "in secret." Only they and their mates know about what they are doing. Midrelationship, they'll come to me seeking advice on how to tell their friends and family of their plans that go against their tribe's value system. Or they are asking me how to handle the hostility, fear, and anger from their tribe after they've announced their plans.

What I'm about to say may seem a bit harsh, but I'm not one to tiptoe around, so I'm just going to say it. The desire to announce your plans to your loved ones, who you know are going to be averse, is just your ego seeking validation or your doubts wanting confirmation. Either way, it's self-serving. Before you even open your mouth to them, deep down you know it won't support your higher good. In an ideal world, you should be shouting from the rooftops what your plans are in this defining and pivotal time in your life, and your loved ones should be cheering you on. But if you know you are going to get negativity from others by disclosing your plans, then don't. Seek support elsewhere. It's not worth it.

> *All we need is clarity of intent. Then if we can get the ego out of the way, the intentions fulfill themselves.*
> *—Deepak Chopra*

Some contend that in order to keep their choices private from well-meaning fearmongers, they would have to lie. This, of course, I don't advocate. Lying is a very fake, destructive way to be, especially when you are pregnant. You do not have to lie.

To put this in perspective, I often ask people if they announce the details of their finances or sex life to their loved ones. Of course they say no. Do they consider this lying? Of course not! Who would? They consider that aspect of their life private, sacred, and no one else's business. The same holds true for your birth plans. If others suspect that your choices are contrary to their tribal beliefs, you've done something to elude your birth plans and there's part of your ego you need to put in check. Should they ask you a pointed question that you do not want to reveal the answer to, just tell them that the answer is something you've decided to keep private or just between you and your significant other. I've seen a lot of celebrities lately tactfully dodge personal questions this way, certainly you can do it, too.

"So, where are you having this baby?" one would ask.

"You know, I've been asked that a few times, and I'm so impressed that people have been so respectful and understanding when I tell them that we are keeping that information private!" you respond.

See how I did that? You assume the best of them (people like that) before they are even given a chance to respond. I've done this a lot of times with people asking when my due date was. Due dates . . . that's a whole other book to be written. I learned early on, though, that people knowing my 40-week due date was *not* an advantage to me, given that I don't follow the typical induction routines. Another point of distress was when people would ask me what names I was considering for the baby. Once, I excitedly shared what we were thinking of naming our baby if it was a boy, and was immediately convinced never to do it again when I got the response, "Sounds like a dog's name." Thanks, I'll be sure to let you know when I think the name you've chosen for your sweet, precious bundle of joy sounds like a word you'd use to describe unsavory bodily functions. I've bitten my tongue at least three times when a child's name is the same as a birth term!

My point? There are just some things you can keep private. Certainly your birth plans are one of them. Although, I do like to make a game of this. For example, to the question, "Where are you having your baby?"

- I was going to squat under the tree the baby was conceived by in Mount Charleston.
- I was thinking that the back seat of my car is quite roomy.
- We're webcasting it, so our producer is picking the right location.

To the question, "When is your due date?"

- In two days (if I'm in first or second trimester), don't I look good?
- On Christmas (or pick the holiday that is farthest away; people have a hard time with the math).
- I have a month window between . . . (Take your 40-week due date and add one month.)
- A month ago. (This one you get the greatest reactions with. The looks are priceless.)

To the question, "Is it a girl or boy?"

- We were just hoping for a human baby. You never know with us.

Honestly, if you are lighthearted and joke about it, people usually let it go and it's an easy way to divert the question.

But for those closer to you, I know you will get pinned down, in which case you just make it clear that the question isn't being discussed. Yes, I know, it will drive them crazy and they may not be happy with you, but oh well. And there will be plenty of time for discussing things afterward. In all likelihood, though, there will be very little discussion afterward. By the time the baby is here and everyone is healthy and happy, others' fears are gone, because you have already stepped through their fear and come out the other side the better for it. It's hard to argue with success. Occasionally there will be some slight discord, but more often than not, the waters are calm and carefree.

I am fortunate that my family tribe falls into the category of supporting my decisions in birth. I always felt safe sharing my plans with them, even though my family runs the gamut of home births to planned C-sections. I so love and appreciate that about my family tribe, and it's given me a template on how to respond when someone does choose a birth route that runs counter to peaceful birthing. This is why I am especially sympathetic toward my clients who aren't afforded that support in their immediate tribe. It prompts me to do what I can to help them find a substitute support system.

My point in delving into this? You are going to have this baby. *You* are. Not your mother, not your sister, not even your husband. *You* are the one who has to live with *your* choices the rest of your life. But, your baby does, too. Don't compromise, or you *will* regret it.

I had one mom in my class who, to appease her husband's fears, chose a birth experience that was the complete opposite of her dreams. It was a mess. Of course, wouldn't this sacrifice—of her dreams, her health, her body, and risking her baby's health—wouldn't this ensure that she'd always have his loyal devotion? After all, she's given him so much, she's proved her loyalty to him, right? Of course he would reciprocate. Shouldn't their future parenting dilemma's and marriage be a cakewalk from here on out? Of course not, and in fact, quite the opposite happened.

I later found out that they divorced. And her biggest regret? Offering herself, her dream, and her baby's health up on the altar of "compromise." There was no compromise here. There were decisions made with false hope and built on lies, all masked beneath the word compromise. There is no compromise in birth. You either stay true to your authentic self, or give up your power for one little thing here and one little thing there until your birth resembles very little of what you felt it should've been. If you give me this, I'll give you that:

- If you agree to internal fetal monitoring, I'll let you hold your baby right after the birth.
- If you have the baby in the hospital this time, I'll think about a home birth next time.
- Just do a C-section this time. We can think about a VBAC if we ever have another.

These trades are what people call "compromise." Giving up your power and choosing what you know to be right because you want to avoid a fight or appease your partner will only put you and your baby's safety in jeopardy and will put you at odds with yourself.

Birth decisions hold as much weight as does trying to decide who to marry. Would you ever consider the following?

- If you marry me (even though you really don't love him), I promise I will make you happy.
- In the prenuptial agreement, if you agree to stay married to me for 10 years than you will get $1 million.
- Just marry this guy so he isn't deported. You can always marry for real in the future.

Nothing kills a growing seed faster than denying your true self and the gut feelings you have. Suppressing what you know is right and then becoming a martyr about it and calling it compromise so that you look like the bigger person? Don't do it. To gain a peaceful birth, you cannot do what is "good enough," you have to decide to do what you feel is best. You cannot have a peaceful birth if the decisions you make only feed your ego or insecurities and not your higher self and path.

"Well, I wanted to do X-Y-Z, but my OB just flat out refused, and my husband talked me into it so that I wouldn't rock the boat too much. I mean, in the long run, it's really no big deal, right?"

If you want a vaginal birth, but your spouse is insisting on a Cesarean and you go ahead with a Cesarean, where is the compromise? Go ahead and insert any item for the words *vaginal* or *Cesarean* in the previous sentence there seems to be a conflict over. You may be willing to offer yourself up as a sacrifice, but are you really willing to compromise your baby's physical, emotional, and spiritual health just to gain someone else's approval? It's selfish and foolish to do so, for all parties. Be mature, be an adult, and be true to yourself and what you know you need to be doing. Yours may not be the popular decisions, and they may not be the easiest at the time, but in the long run your peaceful decisions will be your safest.

> Life only demands from you the strength you possess.
> —David Hammarskjold

    You can get what you want and still be kind and respected. Never, never defend your choices. If they are the right choices for you, they need no defending. Do not argue points with people. This is most easily done the more time you have before your due date and when you're not actually in labor; regardless, it can be done at any time. Tell them that you understand their fears, and that in one month's time you will convene with them again to revisit and see if the meditating and research *they've* done in that time has produced any results. But, let me drive the following home: It is *not* your job to convert them to your way of thinking. It is not your job to make sure they are on the same page as you. They have to make their choices on their own. If they sincerely want to raise themselves to match your frequency, they will. If they aren't sincere, no amount of studies, books, arguments, or "proof" coming from you will change them. You will have wasted your time and energy. In fact, it will likely make them dig their heels in deeper. The burden is on them to plead their case; there's no reason why it should rest solely on you. Forgive them and be grateful for them and their love for you. It is far more powerful to take that approach in order to inspire faith. To understand this principle more, I suggest you read the book *Power vs. Force* by David R. Hawkins.

    If you choose to "compromise," understand that you need to own that decision and not blame anyone else for it. Don't assign your choices to your caregiver's or birthplace's policies or your partner's insistence. Your choices are your choices. Ultimately, it is you and your baby who have to live with your choices.

    Again, be aware that if you are going to commit to a peaceful birth, you cannot afford to engage in an argument or surround yourself with doubters. Moving on, by seeking out support and guidance, does not mean that you are leaving your loved ones behind or rejecting them at all. This process of peaceful birthing can take literal and figurative strength, which only comes in and through love and support. Anything less weakens you. There are people out there waiting to help you. Find them.

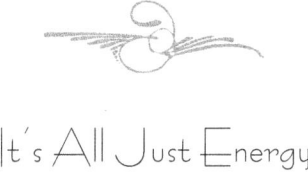

## It's All Just Energy

It's of utmost importance that those attending your birth be loving and supportive and have no agenda but that. I can't tell you how profoundly the energy of just one person can shift the flow and direction of a birth, positively or negatively. And then if you add another person's energy equal to the previous person's energy, well, you get the picture.

Some women invite people to their births out of obligation. Some are invited so that the birthing mother can "teach" or "show" them the way to peaceful birth. And still others fear that without the support of someone in particular they will fail. All of these reasons are rooted in the destructive energy of fear or ego.

When you choose your birth team members (including your caregivers)—your birth tribe, so to speak—be clear that you are choosing them for one reason only: because you love them and they love you. It's that simple.

Close your eyes and bring up an image of all those you've chosen to attend you. Your doctor. Your midwife. Your husband. Your sister. Your friend. Your mother. Your mother-in-law. The energy of your birthplace. Is there anything uneasy or negative that flows through you when you do this?

If so, you have two choices. You can un-invite them or replace them, or you can forgive them and do what you can to inspire them to be on the same page as you and cross your fingers that their presence will be positive.

Let's explore the first option of uninviting or replacing them. I get that this path can be everything from awkward to seemingly impossible to do. Let me assure you that it's not as difficult as you think it is or want it to be. If it's your caregiver who's out of line with your peaceful birth, then switch caregivers. You may say, "Oh, okay, just switch huh? So easy, eh?" Honestly, I've heard every excuse in the book:

1. I'm too far along.
2. I don't have the money.
3. There's no one better.
4. I would hurt their feelings.

I will address each of those points directly.

1. *I'm too far along.* My midwives would always say, "It's not too late to switch until the baby's head is out." I've had multiple clients switch caregivers the day before labor and others switch care even while in labor. To say it's too late is not a viable excuse.
2. *I don't have the money.* So, the caregiver you want isn't covered under your insurance? You don't have the funds? For all five of our births we have paid for them out of pocket, and those pockets had gaping holes, so we've always had this dilemma every single birth. Somehow, it always got worked out and I always got the birth I worked toward.
3. *There's no one better.* If you truly can't find a caregiver to meet your needs in your area, start looking outside your area. Before I got pregnant with our third, we thought we might be living in the Philippines for a short time and I anticipated having a baby while there. I started doing as much digging as I could to find out my options. What I uncovered didn't look attractive in the least. I mean, it was terrible. Those poor Filipino women. I asked my midwives if they'd be willing to fly to the Philippines for three weeks around my due date. They jumped at the thought! In fact, they were a little disappointed when we ended up staying put. Believe me, where there's a will there's a way.
4. *I would hurt their feelings.* This one kills me. Unless you have a personal relationship with your caregiver outside the clinic (and I mean a friendship), the odds of

your hurting their feelings is quite slim. Doctors have clients move, or change insurance coverage all the time, Do you think they are up at night lamenting about it? And if a caregiver is mature and secure, he/she is going to want you to have a caregiver who fits your needs best and won't be hurt that you switched anyway. I've had plenty of loved ones hire a doula other than myself, and I make it crystal clear that I am totally fine with that. After all, it's not about me at all, and if they feel that another doula fits their needs better, I want what they want to achieve their goals. The last thing you should be doing is playing babysitter to other people feelings, especially not your caregiver's.

But let's say it's your mother or sister who wants to be at the birth but you don't want them there. Very rarely has the following statement not fit the bill: "We really thought/meditated/prayed on who should be there and just have a strong feeling that it should only be X, Y, and Z." If they get offended or put out, it's not someone who should be there anyway, because this indicates that they're put their feelings above yours to begin with. A more passive way to approach this is to just not call them when you're in labor. Unless you live with them, you do not need to notify them of anything. You can tell the whole world they are invited to your birth, but unless you call them to come, they aren't going to be there. I actually encourage you to just be authentic and up front and tell them directly, but if that would cause unnecessary stress at a vulnerable time, taking the passive route is valid. A relationship where you can't be up front and still be respected has deeper issues than can be adequately addressed during the short time that pregnancy allows and is an indicator that the relationship would not serve your highest good in labor anyway. If it is your husband or partner you feel should be absent from the birth, my heart goes out to you. This is a delicate situation. Handle this as best you can, but trust that if you stay in a place of peace, faith, and love that all things will work together for your highest good. Whether he voluntarily chooses to remove himself, is unavailable when you go into labor, or that his attitude softens by the time your body surrenders to your baby's coming, I have seen these situations where the partner was not welcome in the birth experience and timing unfold amazingly well.

Maybe you have an excuse as to why you can't have your dream birth team that I didn't address. Whatever your excuses, more than likely it is you who is unwilling to make the hard choices and do the work necessary to shape your birth the way it should be. Choose today to let go of your excuses and take one step forward, and then another tomorrow.

Now let's explore forgiving and being grateful. This path is not always realistic to navigate because you cannot control others. If you feel strongly that you should have people at your birth who don't fully support you, or they embrace their fears or aren't on the same page as you, work daily on visualizing them in a countenance of love and acceptance and faith at your birth. This tool can be extremely powerful. Visualize it, and then, like with all desires, let go of your need for it. Verbally say, *I forgive you of your weaknesses and shortcomings and have faith in your love.* Be grateful for them and their acts of service toward you, then act as if they already support you and visualize yourself connecting with them figuratively and literally. Then trust that that desire will be fulfilled, whether it's by them or through someone else. Through these efforts—faith and surrendering—your needs and desires will likely be met, often in unexpected ways, and maybe better than you could have envisioned.

If you aren't in a place of peace and trust with your birth team, this conflict may manifest itself during labor. Most of the time it shows up in the form of a stalled labor, a baby not descending, maternal or fetal distress, going far past 42 weeks, or a breech or malpositioned baby.

The typical Hollywood depiction of a woman unexpectedly lashing out and verbally abusing her husband during labor and birth is incredibly far from reality. It's never unexpected and can always be predicted by someone who knows how to spot the red flags. That lashing out is just a symptom of a bigger problem in a marriage. A couple doesn't check their core problems at the door once labor begins; rather, they bring them with them, and they can be magnified during this defining moment. It's one of my strongest admonitions for couples. Resolve your big problems before labor begins. Enter into the birth experience with a clean slate. If you do not, and choose to have your mate at the birth anyway, then at least be real with yourself and own the fact that you are letting your ego trump you and your baby's health and wellbeing. That energy can be dangerous in a birth, not to mention just plain heartbreaking to witness what should be the most bonding of experiences become polluted.

I always cringe a bit when a client tells me that her mother, sister, or best friend is flying in for the birth. The odds of her waiting to go into labor until this guest leaves to go back home is high, in my experience. And if the guest is staying until the baby shows up no matter what? Well, the options of induction and talk of scheduled Cesarean come into play, because the woman feels so obligated that she can't relax enough to release adequate hormones to go into or to progress effectively while in labor. That kind of pressure to "perform" is counterproductive. Acceptance and surrender of the timing of the birth, regardless of your agenda, is key to the release of energy and hormones necessary to initiate contractions.

The stress that people or events bring into a labor environment is profound. I remember my childbirth educator recounting the well-documented fact that women who live in war-torn regions actually stop their labors—even near pushing stage—when bombing begins. Ask any doula or midwife and she will tell you that if you feel inhibited by even just one person or the environment you're in, you can stall or completely halt your labor. It's amazing that when certain people, even myself or the caregiver, leave the woman alone and unhindered, how she can finally relax and let her baby come.

So, if you aren't able to forgive and be grateful for those unsupportive people you've chosen to be in your birth team, or if you choose not to ask people to leave during labor or seek out another nurse, OB, or midwife in the midst of labor, accept that you've reduced your odds of achieving a peaceful birth. The word I want to emphasize in that last sentence is the word *you*. You have chosen this, no one else. You are not a victim in this whole experience, and in order to progress during and after the birth as a woman and as a mother, it's essential you take responsibility for your choices and don't feign victimhood, no matter the outcome.

So, in conclusion, improve your thoughts and inner mind chatter and choose the information that you give your tribe carefully.

> *Our deepest fear is not that we are inadequate. Our deepest fear is that we are powerful beyond measure. It is our light, not our darkness that most frightens us. We ask*

*ourselves, Who am I to be brilliant, gorgeous, talented, fabulous? Actually, who are you not to be? You are a child of God. Your playing small does not serve the world. There is nothing enlightened about shrinking so that other people won't feel insecure around you. We are all meant to shine, as children do. We were born to make manifest the glory of God that is within us. It's not just in some of us; it's in everyone. And as we let our own light shine, we unconsciously give other people permission to do the same. As we are liberated from our own fear, our presence automatically liberates others.*

Marianne Williamson, *A Return to Love*

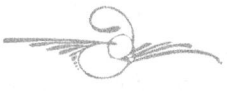

## Just the Facts

When I was pregnant with my first baby, I realized—close to my due date—that we needed to decide what we were going to do about vaccinations.

To be completely honest, I had only the minutest of ideas of what a vaccination was. I had zero feelings on them either way. I don't have a conscious memory of getting a vaccine, although my mom later informed me that my last shot was when I was 5. Never in my life had I heard a discussion about it or read anything on it. For this decision, I was a clean slate, starting from scratch. What a huge advantage! No fear to weed out or myths to debunk.

I did as much research as I could, even though back in 1996 there wasn't a whole lot out there on the subject. I quickly found out what the status quo was and realized that if I were to deviate from the mainstream, that I might encounter some resistance. Beyond that, I didn't think much of it until I started hosting and then taught a vaccination class in conjunction with my childbirth education class.

I decided that teaching the subject would be a piece of cake. I naively assumed that everyone made this decision the same way I made it—gather the facts, make my decision, check in with God to see if He supported my decision, and move on. What is so hard about it?

Very soon after I began teaching the class I realized that the beliefs and fears regarding vaccinating—or better put, *not* vaccinating—were deep and powerful. People found it very difficult to consider that these societal tribal beliefs that had been ingrained in them just might not be true.

"Wait, are you telling me that polio wasn't eradicated because of the vaccine?"[24]

Sometimes I would have to go over just that answer in three or four different ways for them to grasp what I was saying. The logic and facts were there in black-and-white, so it was impossible to argue with, but they just couldn't reconcile it with themselves. It was almost as if I was proving that their god didn't exist. It's usually almost too much to digest—almost. At the end of the vaccination class I encourage people to take the information, meditate or pray about it and make a choice based on what feels peaceful. Never once has anyone come back to me saying they regretted making their decision that way.

This decision about whether or not to vaccinate for most, I discovered, was by and large fear-based and not rooted in facts or logic whatsoever. And that's when I realized I had to incorporate a different approach to teaching my vaccination class. "Just the facts" was not a good enough approach to educating someone on inoculations. And the same goes for many of your birth beliefs.

> "We are not always given the knowledge of what will happen. Graciously, we are given inspiration and the gift of choice is ours."
>
> - Pam Udy, ICAN (International Cesarean Awareness Network) President, 2007-2009

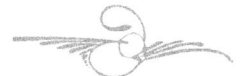

## Ripple Effect

I mention vaccinations because you have things to decide on immediately after the birth, and how you approach them will color your birth experience. Once you get clear on your path and move toward your peaceful birth, something magical happens in all areas of your life. By releasing your negative talk and false beliefs (and resulting destructive behavior) about something this big, ancient and universal, it gives you the ability to effortlessly release your destructive beliefs in multiple areas of your life. And when you do achieve your peaceful birth, it can be one easy way to put the stamp on moving forward in all areas of your life and striving for a peaceful way of being. You know what contentment, empowerment, and bliss are. You have raised your frequency. It is up to you to act on this opportunity to grow.

It is difficult in the first three to twelve months postpartum not to seek after that high you experienced at childbirth and replicate it on a consistent, more permanent basis. It becomes clear what areas of your life are not on the same frequency as that of your peaceful birth, and you will have an urge to improve those areas. You will begin to question all those things that make you feel out of sync with peace. After all, if a joyful, peaceful birth is possible—something that the PABC tells us is not frequent or possible at all—than what else is possible? What else in your life is the result of fear, doubt, and control? What other lies have you believed and been telling yourself?

You may begin to effortlessly attract interactions and people into your life that match your new frequency; that of peace, love, faith, contentment, health, and progress.

This ripple effect truly is amazing. It will impact the way you parent, feed, nurture and educate your child. It will improve your relationship with yourself and those around you. It will allow your greatest good to flow to you—*if* you pay attention and actively work on moving toward that space.

Certainly you can do all this work of having a peaceful birth and leave it at that. And honestly, that's great in and of itself. You could choose to abandon this mindset the day after the birth and suppress that small voice inside you telling you to parent and live authentically and without strife. But that would be sad, wouldn't it?

You can do it. And guess what? It may just be easy, and it will definitely be worth it. As you begin to listen objectively to all the beliefs you tell yourself or that others tell you, ask yourself if it's something worth holding onto or if the opposite belief is something worth exploring. As you begin doing this, it may be hard at first to illuminate those programmed beliefs, but eventually it will become second nature the more you practice doing it. Weeding out those mindsets that don't serve you will become a piece of cake. It is awesome to know that you are the creator of the kind of birth you want, the parent you become, and the life you live.

The following are common parenting beliefs. As you read them, ask yourself if it's a belief you hold, and if the reason you believe it is rooted in fear or love. Then choose if you want to continue to structure your life around that belief.

1. Do you believe that breast-feeding has to be hard, painful and inconvenient?
2. What are your feelings about breast-feeding in public? Do you believe a breast-feeding couple should be hidden away or completely covered, or is nursing in public something that can be tactfully navigated?
3. Do you feel that breast-feeding past 3, 6, 9, 12, 18, or 24+ months is weird and spoils the baby, or do you trust that you and the baby will know when the healthiest time to completely wean is?
4. What do you believe about sharing a bed with your baby? Do you believe that bed sharing is dangerous and leads to unhealthy sexual behaviors, an over-dependant and spoiled child, or that it would negatively impact your sex life with your mate? Or do you espouse the belief that gentle parenting also extends into the night, and that your families needs may be best met by possibly sharing a bed?
5. Do you think holding a baby often, even all day, creates an over-dependant and spoiled baby? Or that a baby can never receive too much love and affection and will be more secure and independent the more they are shown the love you have for them?
6. Is it good to get a baby used to a bottle, pacifier, or crib

so they can detach from you more easily? Or are you more confident in allowing unhindered access to you so you can get to know your child's needs better?
7. Do you believe that a detached parent/child relationship is a healthy relationship?
8. Do you think other people know more about the health and safety of your baby than you? Or do you feel confident that you can gather all your resources and make the best decision possible for your child?

The other day I was driving by the Red Cross mobile blood bank motor home. My 7-year-old asked me what it was. To reply, "People go in there and other people take their blood" just didn't seem like it would evoke a very good image of the purpose of the motor home. So, I decided to do the lengthier explanation.

"Well, sometimes people need operations if they are in a car accident or something, and in order to do an operation you need extra blood to give to that person so they heal better. So people go in there, and the nurses in there stick a needle in your arm to take out some of your blood so they can save it for when someone needs an operation."

"Oh. Can anybody give their blood?" she asked

"Well, most everyone, but your blood needs to match the person having the operation, so people who have 0+ blood should give blood all the time, because most people have that type of blood," I could hear myself midsentence and realized I had probably completely lost her on the whole blood type thing.

She sat in contemplation and then said, "I'm oh so positive I could give them my blood."

"Yes, baby, you are oh so positive," I said laughing, "but wait till you're a little older so you have more blood to give."

Early on in my doula career, I would watch a TV show that would follow a woman or couple through the last few weeks of their pregnancy, through the birth, and a snapshot of the postpartum, all in 30 minutes. You know, reality television - haha. I would try to catch and record the nice births to show snippets in my childbirth education classes, but very few of the births were peaceful ones.

More often than not, I'd get sucked into watching all the drama-filled births. The lady who wailed at 1 cm and wouldn't stop no matter what kind of support she got, the lady who insisted on calling everyone by their first *and* middle names—even her doctor; the lady who only planned a C-section because she wanted to accommodate her doctor's, husband's, and mother's schedules; the one who thought a natural birth must be easy so why plan for anything. Oy! I could predict with 97 percent accuracy how the birth would end up from the first two minutes of the episode. Yet I'd still sit there, building up my irritation, becoming more jaded and cynical, and the show would culminate with me yelling at the TV screen, telling the parents why this or that happened and how they could have avoided what they were complaining about.

One day I overheard my oldest daughter, then 4 years old, telling her friend, "My mom is always yelling at the TV. I don't know why." That's when I knew I had a problem. Hello. My name is Amy, and I like to involve myself in other people's dramatic births. There is no 12-step program for this one.

Once I eliminated that one behavior, my clients' births were markedly more smooth and enjoyable. I didn't realize how much this one, seemingly benign activity was leaving me feeling anxious and defensive at births. None of it helped me, my clients, or the others in the birth team.

In life, especially during pregnancy, you have to surround yourself with friends, family, reading material, and media that support and share your views and philosophies in order to achieve and maintain your goals.

It's okay to be in the world, just not partaking of the predominant destructive tribal mentality. One way to do that is to understand that most of those around you are not on the same playing field. In fact, they don't even know a game is being played, much less able to locate the field where you are.

> Some tribes are stuck. They embrace the status quo and drown out any tribe member who dares to question authority and the accepted order. . . . They create little value and they're sort of boring.
> —Seth Godin, *Tribes*

I have been so very fortunate to have great tribes. Shortly before I decided to become a doula and childbirth educator in 1996, we moved back to my hometown of Las Vegas. I wrongly assumed there would be a doula and childbirth educator association already formed for me to just step into, like there was where I delivered my first baby. I looked in the phone book for doulas and childbirth educators. There was nothing. Back then, the Internet was of no help in this department, so I thought I'd cold call some midwives in the phone book to see if they knew of anything. I got everything from, "Oh, yes! I've heard of doulas! But I don't know of any here" to "Now tell me, what are doulas?" I was a bit discouraged. I contacted some childbirth training organizations and got the names of two women in my area who were teaching childbirth education. I asked each of them if there was a group. Nope. Then, for some odd reason, I asked them if I formed a group, would they come to meetings. They were totally up for it. Therein began Childbirth Educators and Labor Assistants of Southern Nevada. The group grew from the three of us, to over 25 when I stepped down as president 11 years later. During that time, one of my childbirth education students asked me if there was a mom's group she could join. I really knew of none, but I thought, "Hey, why not start one?" So, I did. We started off with about 10 members and at our peak had about 150 amazing members. It's still a thriving, great group today! My point is, if there isn't a group already formed, there's no reason why you can't start one yourself. Having a support group of likeminded women is powerful.

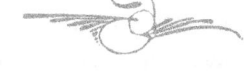

## Be Happy Now: Stepping Out of the PABC Mentality Today

One of the easiest ways to move tribes and increase the odds of achieving your peaceful birth is to be happy now, right this second. I know, I know. We are all told that pregnancy is horrible, full of this and that problem. We are expected, even encouraged to complain and bemoan ourselves. It's our one trump card that no one can take from us, right?

"Man, my back hurts," your husband complains.

"Oh, yeah? Try carrying around 30 extra pounds that pinch your nerves and then you can complain."

Let me suggest something plainly. Stop it, and become grateful right now. If you want to pull happiness and peace into your birth, start with your pregnancy and be happy now. Yes, you may have hemorrhoids that would put a cluster of grapes to shame. Yes, your feet may look like stuffed sausage. Yes, you can fill an Olympic-sized swimming pool with your urine output. So what? Do you *want* to feel that way? Do you really think that complaining about it is going to relieve it?

Do you know someone, maybe even yourself, who is is the ultimate martyr for the cause? The minute she finds out she's pregnant, it starts. She's just so sick, so tired, every smell, color, or look bothers her. Then it becomes her unbearable back pain, leg cramps, varicose veins, she looks so fat, she has heartburn. The maladies she can complain about are never ending. And of course, she's the only one who has ever felt that way. The only other people who can stand to be around her are those with the same mentality; other pregnant women who are looking to compete with her and one-up her complaints. Lucky for her, they aren't hard to find. Yeah, that's a fun tribe to be a part of. Where *don't* I sign up?

When my pregnancy test confirmed my third pregnancy, I made a conscious choice and effort. I was going to enjoy this pregnancy. Even if I had swollen sausage feet like I had before (which I did), debilitating heartburn (which I did), food aversions (who doesn't?) and back pain, I was going to be a pregnant goddess and enjoy this pregnancy.

Whenever someone would ask how I was feeling, I'd respond with conviction, "Like a goddess!" whether I did or not. The reactions I'd get were always great. And while that pregnancy wasn't devoid of all discomforts, I remember it being easier than my first two, for sure. All I really remember, emotionally speaking, from that pregnancy was a lot of joy and fun.

Discomforts will likely happen, but misery is optional. Be happy and joyful in spite of the imperfections. Doing this now will help you navigate the discomfort and pain of labor, birth, and postpartum. Because if you are waiting for your pregnancy to be discomfort-free before you are happy with it, you will wait your entire nine months away.

Go ahead and write down all your complaints, those phrases you repeat over and over. Are they one of these?

- *I'm so fat.*
- *I'm so hot.*
- *I pee all the time.*
- *I can't get a good night's rest.*
- *I'm ugly.*
- *When is this going to be over?*
- *This baby is beating me up.*

Come on, what are they? Write them here.

_____

_____

_____

_____

_____

_____

_____

_____

_____

Go ahead and feel it, be sorry for yourself. Now, say what you wrote down out loud for the last time. Then let it go. Release it.

You are now:

- Beautiful
- *Healthy*
- *Radiant*
- *Comfortable*
- *Functioning optimally*
- *Sleeping perfectly*
- *Enjoying every minute you get to spend growing and nurturing your baby*
- *Loving your baby, and your baby loves being a part of you.*

Below, replace any negative phrase you wrote down with the opposite, positive affirmation.

_____

_____

_____

_____

_____

_____

_____

_____

_____

You have all the right body parts and health in place to conceive and carry a baby. You have the strength and endurance to nourish yourself and grow another human being. Aren't you in awe of this miracle? Just because pregnancy and birth is common doesn't make it any less miraculous. You are a participant in something unique and, frankly, incredibly awesome and beautiful. Your pregnant body is beautiful. Your baby is a miracle. Be happy, be grateful, be amazed! What an honor to carry another life in you. You can grow limbs and organs and a nervous system and connect with your baby in a way no one else can. That is amazing! What an incredible experience you are having; one which some women desperately want but can never have. You are a creative goddess. Act like it!

If you didn't do the last exercise, why not? Are you scared that if you let go of your pain you won't recognize yourself? You are not your pain and you are not your fear. You are already powerful beyond measure. And hanging onto your pain prevents you from accessing that power. Are you afraid to be powerful and happy? If you aren't willing to let go of your addiction to self-loathing and gripes, how in the world do you expect to enjoy your birth experience?

The next minute, the next hour, the next day is determined from this moment. Why not put out there what you want to get back? So many people say they want a good birth experience, but they aren't always willing to do what they need to get it. Don't be one of those people. This energy is like a boomerang. You get what you give. If you give grief and discomforts, that's what you'll get. If you give gratitude and love, that's what you'll get. It's your choice. You are not a victim.

## Extraordinary Births and Peaceful, Unexpected Outcomes

Knowing what is possible and witnessing how others deal with the unexpected help us to shed harmful myths we've carried around with us, sometimes our whole lives, about being female, pregnancy, birth, breast-feeding, mothering, and what is healthy. Thus we are empowered to make new choices and embrace the good, no matter the outcome.

## The Story of Emma Sage

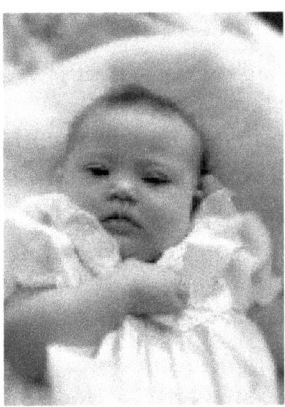

Emma Sage is our fifth child. Early in my pregnancy I began dreaming about a perfect little girl who resembled a china doll. She was so beautiful. Subsequent dreams included a labor and delivery on the side of the road. It would be a recurring theme, a series of dreams, where her labor and birth happened everywhere. My sister, a labor and delivery nurse, brought me a cord clamp and told me to keep it with me, just in case there was a need, as she laughed about all of my stories.

We had no idea that clamp would be used.

We took a family vacation to Florida at about eight weeks. It was during this trip that another powerful sensation overcame me. As we waited for the Blues Brothers to begin their show, I watched a little boy dancing around. He would come up to us, smile, and then dance his way back to his parents. During the show, I could not keep my eyes off him. I looked at Rick and told him that our little one would look just like him. He had a little bit of something extra on his twenty-first pair, by way of Down syndrome. Rick put his arm around me and said, "That would be just fine." I shared this story later with my sister, and then forgot about it.

At my thirteen-week visit, I was measuring big, so I asked my midwife if I could have an ultrasound to rule out twins, Rick agreed. I was actually still so nervous about the pregnancy that I wanted a little peek at our little one. I did not know then that this would actually be one of the worst experiences in my life. As the process began, the technician was cold and seemed rather unconcerned about my comfort. During the middle of the scan, she announced, "There is something wrong with this baby" and then immediately called my midwife. I remember hearing her say, "I think we have a problem."

Instead of having a little peek, relieving me of some stress and reassuring me, this woman sent us on our way feeling scared and confused. We left there and headed straight for our midwife Peggy's office. She told us that the baby's nuchual translucency measurement, the thickness of the skin on the neck, was abnormal. Our baby was measuring at 3.6 mm and anything over 3.5 is considered a soft marker for Down syndrome.

It was a difficult day.

Later that night Rick and I sat outside in the barn on his motorcycle and talked. I was just so scared not knowing what the future held. At one point, I asked, "What are we going to do?" His response, "We are having a baby. We are not God, nor should we ever play God." Oh how I love this man; not only is he my best friend, he also provides strength and support. An amniocentesis was not an option, and we did not want one. We did schedule a level II ultrasound for nineteen weeks' gestation at a hospital near us.

It was the beginning of my quest to find out everything that I could about nuchual translucency, soft markers, and Down syndrome.

The time between that day and the scan at nineteen weeks proved to be enlightening. Everyone who asked me about my pregnancy heard about the possibility that the baby might have Down syndrome and the responses I got amazed me. Some would say things like "you will be truly blessed" others would say, "What are you going to do?" but the responses that were most difficult included "You're not going to have it are you?"

My sister came with me for the level II ultrasound. She was experienced in this department, and I wanted her with me so that she could keep her eyes on the scan—

focusing on the baby's heart and other major organs. The baby was free of any structural defects and the nuchual translucency was no longer an issue. There would be another scan at twenty-eight weeks. The baby had no soft markers for Down syndrome at that time, but I knew in my heart already that she would be born with that extra little chromosome.

I celebrated this pregnancy. I shared the joy with everyone. The possibility of trisomy 21 didn't matter.

This was our baby, our perfect, beautiful baby.

My dreams continued to intensify. At least once a week I dreamt of the baby's unexpected birth and my sister always laughed at my stories about the unusual places the baby was born. I kept the cord clamp with me, as I kept dreaming of an angel—that I thought might have been the baby we lost reassuring me everything was going to be fine.

On my due date, I checked out Babies with Down Syndrome from our local library, along with a bunch of books about gardening. When my mother-in-law saw it she looked at me and said, "You're not going to need this book," I just smiled and said, "I know, it's just in case."

On Tuesday, May 8, three days after she was due, I was helping my daughter with a science project. When it was complete, everyone headed to bed early, as Rick had to leave by 3:00 a.m. I was having a bout of indigestion, and headed downstairs to take a warm bath. After the bath, I felt better and went out to the recliner, and fell asleep. About an hour later, I woke up in pain, and took another bath. This happened three times. The next time I woke up, it was 1:00 a.m. and I thought I might have been having contractions about fifteen minutes apart. I called my sister and told her what was going on; by this time, I was in a great deal of pain. She told me to call my midwife and she would get dressed and meet me at the hospital.

I left a message for the midwife at about 1:25 a.m. and waited for her call. During this time, the contractions seemed to be coming in waves, never really ending, just continuing. When she called back, the phone woke up Rick.

*He jumped out of bed and dressed because he knew something was going on. I told her I was not sure that this was the start of labor, and that I felt so weird. I thought it might be possible that she would check me and send me back home, but we agreed to meet at the hospital anyway. We woke up the children and that was when a contraction that really scared me hit. I managed to get him dressed and then began dressing myself.*

*As I began pulling up my overalls, I got another contraction that hit me like a ton of bricks.*

*I remember thinking that if this was only the beginning of labor I was not going to be able to handle what happened next. I walked down the stairs as Rick and the children were already on their way out the door. Just before I reached the bottom, I had a strong sensation to go to the bathroom. I yelled for Rick, just as I realized this baby was well on its way, and I began pulling off my clothes. "Where do I go?" I asked Rick. I thought maybe the living room or back up to bed, but Rick told me to get into the bathtub, as he threw in a bunch of clean clothes in a suitcase while calling 911.*

*I listened as he asked the children "Kids, quick, what is our address again?" It had changed from a rural route just a few years back and he couldn't remember the new one.*

*All those dreams, they had a meaning, they were my preparation for Emma Sage's birth. I didn't know where she would arrive, but I knew it was just going to be us, and that we weren't going to be at the hospital. Rick helped me deliver her, surrounded by our children. As I raised her to my chest, I looked at Rick and said, "Oh look honey, she does have Down syndrome!"*

*Her birthplace was not only unexpected, it also shared an amazing coincidence. Rick's grandfather died, sitting on a closed toilet in this very space. It was a gateway for souls to enter and leave this worldly place. To honor her great-grandfather Alexander, Emma Sage was given a third name—Alexandra.*

*Her birth was peaceful and joyous, not overrun with medical intervention or invasion. We welcomed her into* this world alone, as a family.

When the emergency team arrived the loaded us into the ambulance, and we were off to the hospital. When we arrived, my sister and midwife were there to greet me. My midwife looked at me, smiling and said, "If it is nothing you can send me home." We laughed aloud as Emma Sage had arrived just fourteen minutes after we talked about whether or not I was in labor.

Most newborn babies go to the nursery, but not our Emma Sage. Because she was born outside of the hospital, she was considered a dirty baby and had to stay with us. I would have had it no other way, because most children with Down syndrome are quickly whisked away from their parents for precautionary medical intervention—not our Emma Sage.

We all laugh to this day about the dirty baby who was born in a bathtub. I knew right away she had Down syndrome and my midwife and sister agreed. Many doctors came to peek at her. Hypotonia made her little body weak and unable to maintain her temperature, so they brought in a warmer for us. She was a quiet, sleepy little one.

I tried nursing her but she was unable to latch on. I began pumping right away, as I didn't want them to supplement with formula. I was going to breastfeed her, as I did all of her siblings, for as long as she wanted to. Those first feedings included a syringe, until she was able to latch, but once she figured it out, she nursed like a champion.

So many other unexpected things have happened since the birth of Emma Sage, so many subtle reminders about the true meaning of life.

Emma: The one who heals.

Sage: One with great wisdom.

Emma Sage, a name that she has lived up to since the before she was born.

—Tara Marie,
www.emma-sage.org

## Thalea's Birth Story

With our history we had a few obstacles to overcome before this birth became possible.

*1993*—My first baby was born via induced vaginal delivery at 9 days past my "due date." A week of prodomal labor, 12 hours active/hard labor and 30 minutes of pushing. She was posterior, but born vaginally.

*1997*—Second baby was born via C-section for posterior brow presentation after induced labor (18 hours of hard labor, at least half an hour of pushing and the OBs trying to turn her head during contractions) at 6 days past my "due date." I had not gone into labor on my own, but had been leaking amniotic fluid for 2–3 days and had a low-grade fever.

*2000*—Third baby was born via scheduled repeat C-section (4 days before my "due date") for breech position that turned transverse upon the opening of my uterus, which required an inverted T-incision by the doctor because the baby got stuck. I had a panic attack (the first of many) while they were closing me up and thought I was going to die and never get to know my baby. That was one of the worst experiences of my life.

When I first discovered I was pregnant with this baby I started seeing CNMs attached to the local hospital and overseen by an OB group. I was told at my first appointment that the midwives would see me for my prenatal care until 34 weeks, upon which time they would transfer me to one of the high-risk OBs due to my C-section history. They never verbalized it, but I had a strong feeling that this meant I would have a C-section before 38 weeks. During one of my ultrasounds it was discovered that my placenta was anterior, adding the concern that it may attach to my scar.

Shortly after that, I found and joined the ICAN (International Cesarean Awareness Network) list and read the research on the ICAN site. I spoke through email to two women who had also had either vertical (classical) or inverted T-incisions. I read Natural Birth after Cesarean by Karis Crawford, PhD, and Johanne C. Walters, BSN, RN. Karis herself had an inverted T-incision and went on to have two VBACs. In the midst of this research I decided to find a home birth midwife or at least a midwife that was not working for a hospital/OB group. There was only one in my immediate area that I could locate and she would not assist me. I did a search for home birth midwives on the Internet for my area. There were very few and they either turned me down or didn't return my call. Ohio is apparently fairly unfriendly to lay midwives or Direct Entry Midwives (DEMs) and all Certified Nurse Midwives (CNMs) seemed to be under the thumbs of the OBs and hospitals. So, I expanded my search into Michigan, which luckily is a bit more midwife-friendly. I was still turned down by every midwife within 30–45 minutes of my home. I finally found a DEM-owned birth center nearly 50 miles from my home. We discussed my history and current situation with the anterior placenta, and she said they would be happy to assist me, that they had assisted with other VBAC's after incisions like mine! At 22 weeks I transferred care to the Michigan midwives and began the 45-minute drives to my prenatal appointments.

My pregnancy went along fine, no complications. I was fully planning on giving birth to my daughter at their birth center, but I was prepared for the possibility that I might end up with another C-section due to whatever unforeseen emergent circumstances might arise.

One evening in my 36th week I began having fairly regular contractions, and during these contractions the baby started to flip. I immediately stopped her, believing that she was already vertex. I put my hand against whichever part it was and pushed it back to the top of my belly. At 37 weeks the midwives both felt that the baby was breech upon palpation. They explained that as long as she was in a frank breech position they would still assist me with a VBAC. I, however, was in shock. This was the same road that led me to my last C-section with the inverted T-incision and laying on the table thinking I was going to die. I did not want to repeat that experience. I was angry with myself for stopping her from turning the week before and angry with her for being in that position. I spent that weekend doing everything known to man in an attempt to turn the baby, ice on the top of my belly, pulsatilla, music at the bottom of my belly, hands-and-knees position with my shoulders down, chiropractic, tried to find an acupuncturist with no luck, manual manipulation, you name it. I did get her to a transverse position, which was a start, but I explained to the baby that she couldn't stay their either because that was worse! I did get her back to a vertical position but wasn't sure if she was breech or vertex. I stopped my turning attempts just in case she was vertex. I located a local office that does "reassurance" ultrasounds and made an appointment for the following Saturday. During the ultrasound she was frank breech oblique, with her butt sitting on my left hip and one of her hands was near my cervix. This position was not optimal either. I began the turning techniques again, but not as vigorously. I came to a place of peace with either position being okay as long as there were no limbs or umbilical cord in the way. My fiancé and I talked to the baby a lot, explaining that it would be much easier for both of us if she were to turn head down. She did a lot of turning back and forth in the last few weeks and I had a lot of prodomal labor (several weeks) to show for it.

At my last prenatal appointment, I was 41 weeks 4 days, dilated to 1 cm and 20 percent effaced. Hadn't really had too many contractions the last few days. One of the midwives felt that the baby was vertex again, but I was still trying to be prepared for any eventuality. We went to a relaxing Summer Solstice celebration that evening; everyone wished us good labor energy.

Friday morning around 3:30 am (the same time I'd been waking up nightly for the last 4–5 weeks), I woke up having some good, strong contractions lasting about a minute or longer, about 5–7 minutes apart. They kept me up for an hour or two and then I was able to sleep for a few hours. I was a little disappointed when I woke up that I'd slept so long; I thought for sure it was another false alarm. I stayed in bed most of the day resting and contracting; [the contractions] gradually got stronger, but after dinner slowed down to about 10 minutes apart. I had already talked to one of the midwives a few times, and she suggested that maybe they were giving me a break so I could get some rest and they would pick up again tomorrow. I did sleep pretty well that night and they did pick back up around 3:30 a.m. Saturday. A little stronger than before.

By 10 a.m. they were requiring some attention and were starting to hurt. Around 10:30 a.m. I had a very strong one that reminded me how badly labor hurts. A friend of mine, who is a massage therapist, came over after noon and gave me a wonderful back and shoulder massage. By 2 p.m. my contractions progressed; they were 5ish minutes apart, about 1 minute to 1 and a half minutes long and getting continuously stronger. At some point the contractions started hurting in my butt cheeks, which was new to me. My labors with my first two labors involved back labor, but low back, not butt cheeks.

By 6 p.m., I was having difficulty carrying on a conversation during the contractions and they were beginning to require a bit of concentration to get through. I called the midwives and explained my progress as best I could. I was still feeling pretty good but felt like I should be closer to the birth center. She told us to come up and she'd at least check me. That was the most painful car ride of my life! Having strong, painful contractions while on bumpy I-75 and sitting upright! Sheesh! I think I should have sat in the back so I could sit however I wanted. Our midwife met us at the birth center, my fiancé wanted to start bringing our stuff in, but I told him to wait just in case we weren't staying. When she checked me I was already 100 percent effaced and a stretchy 4 cm! Holy crap! I didn't think I was that far along but thrilled that I was!

Labor continued, my friend, the massage therapist, had come with us. The pain in my butt cheeks quickly became unbearable. At this point I started to go inside myself during contractions, which is what I did during my induced labors. Somehow I decided I didn't want to do that this time, I wanted to be more connected to the people in the room. During my inductions I was not able to connect to anyone else in the room or communicate very well at all. This time I tried to keep my eyes open during contractions and to focus on something, anything in the room. It was extremely difficult, but it did help. Also my friend massaged my hips and butt cheeks during each contraction, that helped make it much more bearable. I'm pretty sure she wasn't counting on having to play with my butt all night. At some point my water broke and the contractions got even stronger. I think within an hour of my water breaking my body started to push a bit with the contractions. I tried really hard not to, I knew I wasn't dilated enough and didn't want to make my cervix swell. It was very hard not to push; my body was pushing on its own. A few hours after that I got in the tub. I labored in the tub for a while before I couldn't fight pushing anymore.

Around 3 a.m. I couldn't not push anymore, it was uncontrollable. Someone went to wake up the midwife, who'd laid down for a quick nap. She came back to check me at 3:30 a.m. and I was at 10 cm!! And the baby was LOA (left occiput anterior—the ideal position to pass through the birth canal)! What luck! With the next contraction I pushed as hard as I could, I think it took me two or three pushes to get Thalea's head past my public bone. Then the ring of fire. Ahh! When I got to that point the midwife asked me to stop pushing so hard, to just do slow, gentle pushes, she wanted me to let my body slowly stretch to let the baby through without tearing. That wasn't fun at all. I did what I could to not push too hard.

Finally, her head appeared, for the first time in four births I was able to reach down and feel my baby as she was coming out. A minute later I tried to reach down to pull her out, but there wasn't enough of her out yet. Everyone knew what I was trying to do and stopped me. Thalea wiggled a few times while she was in the birth canal; that is the most bizarre feeling on the planet. A few more gentle pushes and she was completely out! The midwife had lifted Thalea out of the water and slipped one loop of her umbilical cord off her neck and I reached over instinctively and slipped the second loop off. (Seemed completely natural to me at the time, but a little odd that it seemed so natural later.) I took her from the midwife and laid her on my chest. We were all laughing and talking to her, I checked to make sure that she was in fact a girl.

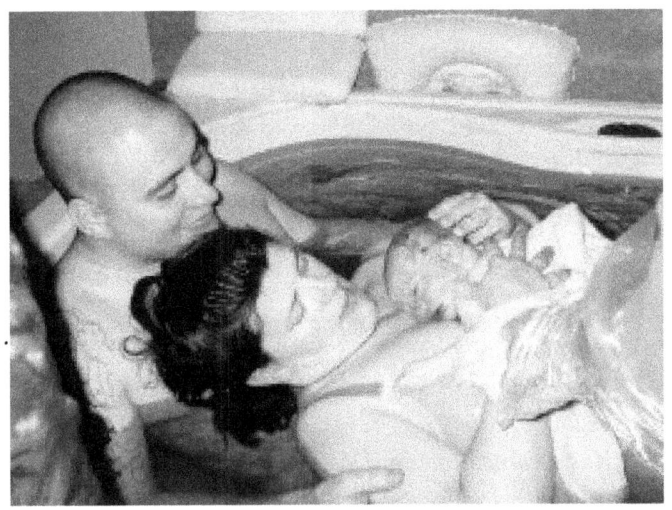

After a few minutes she opened her eyes and started looking around. I birthed the placenta within about 20 minutes or so, without any problems. Daddy was trapped behind me and a little startled that we were sitting in a tub full of blood, amniotic fluid and who knows what else. Finally, it was time to get out of the tub and since I was laying on Tony and the baby was laying on me, Tony decided to let his dad hold her first after me, so we could get out of the tub. Getting out of the tub was quite the chore, but we both had plenty of help. I made my way to the bathroom and then to the bed. The midwife checked me out and no tears! I was quite impressed with this as my first baby was a pound and a half smaller but I did get the obligatory episiotomy at the hospital. Eventually, after everyone got to hold the baby, I got her back and we made our first attempt at breastfeeding. She wasn't terribly interested but she did make a good effort. From the time she was born until this point she'd been wide awake and very alert, but had not cried at all. Our family and friends left around 5 a.m. and we all laid down for some sleep. I didn't sleep much at all, I was too enamored with my new baby girl, I just laid there next to her watching her sleep.

Finally around 10 a.m., Tony got up and got the midwife up. He got our stuff together while I got myself together. It was incredible to be able to stand up and walk to the bathroom unassisted six hours after giving birth and not feeling like I had to hold my guts in! We were home shortly after noon. She had a cone head for a few hours, but it was gone before we even got up to leave from the birth center.

I truly feel like I could not have had this birth without everyone who was there. Had I not had their strength to draw from and lean on during my pregnancy and during my labor, it might have had quite a different outcome.

Thalea Sage, 8 lbs., 3 ozs., 24 inches long with a 14-inch head.

It is so amazing what your body will do, when it's left to its own devices.

—Jessica, www.jessicas-haven.com

## H.M.'s Birth Story

I woke up at 5 a.m. on Tuesday, July 21st, with mild, but consistent contractions. I didn't wake my husband, instead I turned off his alarm and let him sleep. I knew he wouldn't be going to work and I wanted him to get his rest so he could help when the time came. I woke him at 8:30 so that he could go get me something to eat and I told him we'd be having a baby that day and no work for him—he was excited! After he got me breakfast (a bagel and cream cheese) he went back to sleep until 10:15. When he got up the second time we called the midwife and doula to let them know that we'd need them later in the day. He and I labored together for most of the day and Nettie, our doula, came at about 3:30 in the afternoon. At this point I was in the labor pool, relaxing between contractions, which were 3 minutes apart and 1 minute long. The pool was great, too great—it slowed the contractions down. Sooooo, up I got and my husband helped me dress—we took a walk on the rail trail. It was raining during our walk, but it made the contractions come long, hard, and close together—every time I got one he would hold me and help me squat down. The walk made me vomit up everything I had eaten that day, but that's to be expected.

Once we got back to the house things were really picking up and I moved between sitting on the edge of the futon in a supported squat and sitting on the toilet. In fact I was on the toilet when my water broke. One of the funniest things Nettie or I had ever seen was my husband's face when my water broke—it was a huge pop, gush, and splash—he literally jumped! Nettie had to tell him that it was okay, and just my water breaking, not the baby. And in true OCD form, since I was on the toilet there was nothing for anyone to clean up. This is when our midwife showed up, at 8:30 p.m. —just in time, because I was seriously feeling the need to push. Amelia checked me and I was 8 cm!. For the next couple of hours I labored on the birth stool and in the hands and knees position. Finally (or finally as far as I was concerned) I reached 10 cm and was given the go-ahead to push. Pushing was hard, but I loved it; contractions are so much more tolerable when you can actively do something with them, instead of breathing/moving through them. During pushing I was in every position known to woman-kind: hands/knees, side-lying, lunge, modified lunge, squat, supported squat, birth stool, birth sling, walking on the stairs, hands/knees on the stairs. If there was a position to be in, I did it. We literally did it all and it was exhausting.

I started pushing at 10:30 and after two hours Amelia checked me—the baby was at -1 station. I had been at -1 when I started pushing. In fact I pushed for 6.5 hours and the baby never moved past -1 station, which was shocking and disappointing since I was literally doing everything possible. I was not just lying on my back, waiting for the baby to come, I was working her out! My husband was so great, he helped me into all positions, there was even one—the supported squat—where he literally had to hold my full weight plus the force of me pushing. He later said he thought I was gonna take him down. He couldn't believe how strong I was and how hard I was pushing. He got me water and made me drink, he also fed me yogurt and kept trying to get me to eat, he knew I had to keep my strength up and I was getting tired. The midwife finally put in an IV of fluids to get my energy up. She eventually put in a 2nd bag as well, but nothing was helping.

At 5 a.m., after I had been up for 24 hours, he asked the midwife what our other options were because he didn't think I could push forever and we had made zero progress. Amelia suggested the pool or more walking up and down the stairs, but he was on point and asked if she'd ever seen this before and if so, what had that couple done. Amelia told us that she once had a woman push for 8 hours without progress and that that woman had to transfer to the hospital for a C-section. He looked at me and said he thought this was the best plan. I was out of it. I was so tired and had worked so hard and was continuing to have long and hard contractions . . . I knew that he knew what I wanted and that he would only recommend what he thought was really necessary. I agreed to go and told him I wanted to try not to have a C-section. He let the dogs out, helped me get dressed, and grabbed our emergency hospital bag (I packed one in advance, just in case). Amelia called the hospital to tell them that we were coming in. I want to mention that this was not considered an emergency transfer, because neither I nor the baby were in any distress, our heart rates/BP were fine. In fact, the baby labored really well—her heart rate never dropped and she was kicking/punching during the whole labor, which only made the contractions more intense!

We drove to the hospital (15 minutes away) and checked into Labor and Delivery. I was still pushing, it is impossible to stop that force in your body. The nurse was yelling at me to stop pushing while I was in the wheelchair—I completely ignored her. After 6.5 hours of pushing with no progress, I didn't think pushing those last few minutes was going to bring the baby, and if it did, well yay for me! The nurses in L&D were awesome. In fact my nurse was a Certified Professional Midwife who had had all her kids at home. She told me I was doing a *great job but that I had made the right choice to come in. They did an ultrasound on the baby (our first the whole pregnancy) and couldn't see the baby because my bladder was in the way. The IV fluids the midwife put in, well they never came out, and my bladder became distended, pushing on my uterus. They put in a Foley catheter and drained over 32 oz of fluid; that made me feel a lot better! The OB checked me and said that a C-section was the only way to go. The baby was in the posterior position (the back of her head pressed against my back) and that her head was stuck above my pelvic bone. He said he could let me keep pushing, but that 6.5 hours was a lot of pushing and no progress was a sign that something wasn't right. He was concerned that if I did manage to pass her head then her shoulders would get stuck and then that would be an emergency. I asked if an epidural or Pitocin would help—the doc said I didn't need Pitocin since I was fully dilated and that the epidural might make me more comfortable, but that I would still have to get her head unstuck. Pushing with the epidural would be less effective than the pushing in various upright positions I had already done. He let us decide. I love that he didn't dictate or insist. My husband said he thought the C-section was the way to go. I cried and then agreed. It was very quick from there.*

*Up to the OR we went, they put a spinal block in me twice, since the 1st didn't work. Then I was laid back on the table and my husband came in all dressed in scrubs. Minutes later H.M. was out and crying loud—July 22nd, 7:03 a.m. They didn't announce what we had, we asked them to show the baby to my husband and let him announce, which they did. It was awesome—I turned my head and there she was, naked and crying and my husband said—we have a girl, a really big girl! He got choked up and so did I. The OB who did the surgery told me that my next baby would be a VBAC and I was so happy to hear that and to know that he supported it. He said he'd gladly do it, that I clearly had no problem laboring or dilating, just a big girl in a bad position. After the surgery was over* the OB even kissed me on the forehead and told me I did a great job. We feel so lucky that this was the on-call doctor we got.

I told my husband that he had to stay with the baby no matter what. He did. He followed her everywhere and didn't let them do anything but the bare minimum! No eye ointment, no immediate bath, no shots. The hospital staff was very understanding and helpful. I was in recovery for an hour, I did my best to speed through the tests and then I was in maternity and H.M. was with me!

I refused all postpartum medication, with the exception of ibuprofen—I wanted to make sure I was up and aware and that nothing would affect my breast milk. I know they say that the meds don't hurt your breast milk, but I wanted to be extra sure. The nurses and lactation consultant were great—they worked with us on latch at every shift! H.M. was a champ, and we learned together very quickly. The only problem was that since she was born via C-section she has amniotic fluid in her stomach and lungs, so she did a lot of projectile vomiting the first couple of days. Her weight went from 9lbs 5ozs to 8lbs 8ozs. My milk came in full force on Saturday and we've been feeding like mad ever since and her vomiting has stopped.

The doctors wanted to keep me in the hospital until at least Sunday, but I requested an early checkout, I hated being in the hospital. Though the staff was great, being home is always better. We checked out of the hospital Saturday, July 25th. We've been home, enjoying one another ever since. Sleep comes and goes, but I don't mind. I am so completely in love! We have a beautiful little girl, it was a wild ride, but worth it!

—Flo, Connecticut

# 4

## How to Become a Peaceful Birther

> If you don't know your options, you don't have any.
> —Diana Korte & Roberta Scaer
> *A Good Birth, a Safe Birth*

**B**efore we delve into this chapter, I want you to write down right here as many of your deeply held beliefs about childbirth, such as 'birth is painful/joyous' and 'obstetricians are bad/good'.

_____

_____

_____

_____

_____

_____

_____

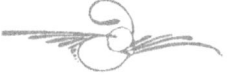

# Lightbulb Moments:
# Personal Enlightenment and Choosing a Guide

There's another aspect to the first night of childbirth class I teach that I love. Since it's a very objective environment and I don't know anyone's background yet, it's the perfect time to present their options to them as a consumer and birthing parent. It's a very safe and nonjudgmental time to do it.

I hang up my large chart, and begin the exercise. I call it "Compare the Caregiver." All the students have a set of cards with "answers" on them that they use to fill in the cell blanks on the chart. I have three columns running at the top of the chart, each labeled *OB, CNM,* and *Midwife (Lay, DEM, CPM)*. The rows going down the left side of the chart are labeled with items such as *C-section rate, mortality rate, cost, philosophy,* and the like. The students proceed to put their answer cards in the cell where they think it belongs. This is a fascinating process to witness. Discussions go on between couples and other students they don't yet really know. Questions start being asked without me having to say a word. They begin to realize that they didn't even know to ask those very important questions that need to be asked to ensure the safest and most satisfying birth possible. They didn't even know they existed. They start to question their assumptions, their tribal beliefs.

After all the cards are placed on the chart, invariably there are cells where there are two or even three cards occupying the space reserved for only one card. I approach the chart, and without explaining or talking, silently move the cards to the right cells. I give them a few moments to study the changes and digest the correct answers. Then one by one I discuss in depth why the answers are what they are. As I do this, it's fun to see the subtle reactions people have as I start to blow one myth after another. A lightbulb here, a lightbulb there. Bling! Bling! Bling! The room starts to illuminate. I love it!

I purposefully do this as the last activity of the night because I want the couples to leave with this new paradigm on their minds. Oh, how I wish I could be a fly on the wall of the car as they drive home! There's a lot of rethinking, a lot of good discussions, maybe some arguments, or a few people convinced that I must be lying or just stupid and wrong.

Whatever the reaction, though, they now know they have choices. They can't play the "I didn't know" card. They know they have viable choices if problems or differences arise in their current situations and they can change things. They know their odds of certain things, like a Cesarean or how much time a caregiver will spend in labor with them. No excuses.

The week between classes is usually a time of enlightenment for them. At the next class, about a quarter of the parents have changed their birth plans or are thinking about changing them.

And, you know what? It was easy to do. Just an open mind and heart, signing up for an out-of-the-box childbirth class, and showing up. It wasn't too hard on my part, either. No, all their questions hadn't been answered, and all their fears hadn't just dissolved, but this exercise illuminates the fact that you don't need to know every little detail in order to take a few steps toward the birth you want. Just trust your gut and those peaceful feelings a little bit. Invite knowledge, truth, and light to help you, and they will.

If everything is in harmony—your heart, your intellect, your faith, your tribe—then you've really got your ducks in a row and your chances of being dissuaded from your peaceful birth are reduced.

But having been in this field since 1997, let me tell you, I can count on one hand how many parents-to-be I've served who have all those ducks lined up and still don't need a guide, a mentor.

Pregnancy puts you in a whole new realm of existence. Women find that they can be affected—physically, emotionally, and psychologically—by things that previously didn't faze them. As much as it can be an incredible time of empowerment and strength, the pendulum can swing the other way, and women can be increasingly vulnerable. Adversities seen and unseen can and will try to play on your weaknesses. It can be very easy to default into old destructive thought patterns, to play scared and overwhelmed and helpless.

There are good odds that most of you have no more than two or three loved ones supporting your birth plans, right? In fact, some of you may have no one—or so you think.

"Hi, my name is Jen, and I got your name from Loretta, a La Leche League leader," the voice on the other end of the phone said.

Now, I didn't know this La Leche League leader and in fact, come to find out, she was across the country. I got this call early on in my doula days, and unbeknownst to me this wouldn't be that last vague call I'd get like this.

"Okay, yes, how can I help you?" I asked.

"Well, I'm due in two months with my second baby. I'm hoping for a VBAC. I've switched OBs three times, and the one I have now just told me he was unwilling to help me do it," she said, a little depressed. At the time, the climate for VBAC was quite favorable, so my immediate thought was, where in the world was she that she ran out of OBs to help her?

She went on to tell me that where she was in Minnesota there were no doulas and she had called around to every OB in town, and no one would even let her get past the word VBAC without shooting her down. She didn't want to give up, though.

"My boyfriend, Tim, is in the military and is stationed at Nellis. I was considering that, if I could find a doctor to support me, and if I could hire you, I could fly out and have the baby there."

Wow. No pressure, right? I start pulling out all my resources because I wanted to see if maybe I knew of a rock she hadn't overturned in her area. What a shame for a pregnant woman to pick up her life and step into a whole new city to get what is rightfully hers. But, alas, there was nothing that I could find.

It looked like her plan of coming to Las Vegas was her best option to achieving a VBAC, even if I was going to be eight months pregnant myself when she was to birth. Had there been another doula in town, I might have referred her on because of the fact that I would be an 8 month pregnant doula, but I was the only doula in town at the time. I asked her if she had a mom, sister, friend, anyone who was helping her out. Nope, just her boyfriend, who was a plane ride away from her.

As she proceeded to tell me more of her story, I realized why she couldn't find an OB to help her. Her initial C-section was a classical incision. This is where, instead of a bikini cut where you are cut into horizontally just above the pubis, you are cut vertically, up and down in the middle of your abdomen. The story she was getting from all of the OBs was that she and her baby would die during labor. She had done her research and knew differently.

She hired me over the phone and we went to work. She was committed to a natural hospital birth. I hooked her up with the one OB in town I knew would have no problems with this. I sent her the educational material she needed, and we communicated often over the next two months.

Two weeks before her due date she flew in. We met in person, crossed all the t's and dotted all the i's. On the day she went into labor, I met them at the hospital, already in labor. It was 6:30 in the morning. Angela was doing the obligatory initial monitoring and had already had an internal exam. Five centimeters and 100 percent effaced. Our first nurse, Gayle, was none too supportive of what was going on. The tension was thick in the room, and she mentioned at least three times in 20 minutes how dangerous this birth was. I did my best to assure her that of course the doctor was supportive and everyone was on the same page. I knew her shift ended at 7:30, so I decided not to invest too much energy or distraction into getting her onboard with us. I just prayed that my favorite nurse, Karen, would take her place.

Imagine my relief when that wish was granted! The hospital was full to capacity that day, and while Angela really wanted a tub in the room to labor in, no such luck. In fact, we got the room that isn't normally used for births unless the hospital was full – it was more of a storage room than a labor room. Even though she was disappointed, she knew that this was something she might have to give up. Angela was doing great, though. The only way I could tell she was having a contraction was if she got really quiet and scrunched her face a little.

Around 8:00 we decided to walk the halls. It was refreshing to see the new sun and know that this baby would be born today. At 9 a.m., Tim decided to run downstairs and get some breakfast while Angela and I went back to the room. She quickly found that sitting on the birth ball was what was most comfortable. Because I'm a big believer in making this as much about the couple as possible, after Tim returned I motioned for him to take my place behind Angela and put pressure on her lower back to relieve the pain. The contractions intensified quickly and I suggested getting in the shower. By 10:00, Angela and Tim were slow dancing in the shower as I directed the showerhead on her back, where she was experiencing most of her sensations. We stayed in there for a good 45 minutes until nurse Karen requested to do an exam. Angela was found to be 8 cm. She was making great, steady progress.

As is normal at this stage, labor picked up and contractions intensified. It was hard for Angela to find a position that worked. She went from side lying, to sitting on the ball, and occasionally squatted next to the bed. When the nurse came in to monitor, Angela mentioned that she was feeling pressure in her bottom. She wanted to go to the bathroom, but accomplishing that was an event. She was hurdling over the hardest part of labor. She had 30 seconds to pee, spent two minutes moaning and rocking at the sink, walked fast to the bed, stopped and moaned and rocked while leaning over the end of the bed for another two minutes. She hurried and knelt on the bed and draped her chest over the birth ball we had put on there. Tim and I rotated massaging her neck and shoulders and applying ample amounts of counter pressure to her lower back. She was moaning and almost crying through these contractions. At 12:15 Karen came in and did an exam. 9.5 cm. Angela quickly got up from lying down and draped herself over the ball again, where her water broke.

Karen was frantically trying to reach the doctor, but Angela was waiting for no one. The urge to push came over her. Angela told me she felt a burning, and I knew full well that the baby was going to be born pronto. The nurse came back and helped us position Angela on her side. Of course by now she was 10 cm, but as is hospital protocol, the nurses encouraged Angela to wait until the doctor came. Tim and I did our best to help Angela slow things down, but it was really a half-hearted attempt on my part. There is no slowing down the inevitable during pushing stage. The baby was born at 1:00 p.m., and the nurses freaked out a little because the baby had a cord around the neck that they had to cut early, but everything was healthy and normal. The doctor showed up five minutes later, completely happy for the couple, and unfazed that he had missed this "high risk, dangerous" birth. Boy, I sure do miss that OB, he was so awesome and trusted birth so much.

The pregnancy went overdue, the birth went textbook, Angela had no medical intervention, not even an IV or hep lock, and she was a classical incision VBAC. Had she given up and succumbed to her barriers, she would have had a scheduled Cesarean. So, when I tell you that you that you may think you don't have support, please believe me when I say to you that you do. There are other women, whether it be moms, doulas, childbirth educators, breast-feeding professionals, that are more than willing to join your tribe. Find them via the Internet, phone book, or asking around. Find them, they are there.

Find them, because you are going to need them. Because, for example, when you are one week overdue, wanting to go into labor spontaneously, and you are "done being pregnant" and your caregiver and loved ones are telling you that it's no big deal to induce—it's safer, easier, and whatever line it is they are feeding you—you will need an objective voice of clarity and reason.

Most women's deepest fear is losing their baby. You're partner's deepest fear is losing you and/or the baby. And honestly, those are a caregiver's deepest fears, too, but maybe for different reasons than what yours are. This fear is played on ad nauseum, not only by health professionals, but also by naysayers in your tribe. When you are tired and worn out and in the midst of a pivotal decision, to hear, "If it were [me, my wife, my baby] I would do XYZ" or "Your baby could die if you make that decision" is a very persuasive argument that can cloud rational judgment in a heartbeat. Even though it's highly manipulative to throw out statements like that, most people believe that the end justifies the means, and if they had to use hard tactics or even lie to you to get you to do what they believe is best and safest, they've done you a favor. It's all with good intentions, but wrong nonetheless.

If you view all parts of yourself as chain links, you begin to understand the meaning of the phrase "A chain is only as strong as its weakest link." If one of your links is weak, in the form of false beliefs, doubtful support people, fears or doubts, it can be that link that breaks the chain to your peaceful birth.

It's important to have people on your team who are knowledgeable, objective, and don't have an emotional or financial stake in the outcome. People to inform you of what your options are, bring your focus back, and point you to the resources you need to make a wise, safe, and peaceful decision.

Of course, I'm not asserting that interventions should always be avoided, but I am saying that you need to be careful, step back, and make a decision that supports your higher spirit, rather than your fear or impatience.

You may still have some fears or destructive beliefs (that you may not even identify as a tribal belief or destructive) that, if played on intensely, especially by an authority figure or someone you seek approval from, can jeopardize not only a peaceful birth, but possibly a safe birth as well. Don't sabotage yourself by denying yourself a personal guide and mentor.

The most common guide is a doula for various and obvious reasons. One, and it's an important one, is because she's objective. Whether your birthplace is home, birth center, hospital, or under a tree on top of a very steep mountain—or whether you birth vaginally, surgically, naturally, or medicated—she has no personal benefit from your birthing in any location or in any way. Secondly, she does become your friend and really does have your best interest at heart. That's why she became a doula in the first place, to help women achieve their goals. She herself understands the importance of this pivotal event and wants to fill that need for you. Only *you* can hire or fire her, so her agenda and allegiance is to you. Additionally, she's educated and experienced. She will not only help you navigate the sometimes unpredictable and possibly choppy waters of labor and birth, but she also serves as a bridge between you and hospital staff. She will help you understand the technicalities of your choices and knows the tools at your disposal to guide your labor along. And she will almost always know of local resources that you can access (e.g., support groups), and also knows tips and tricks of the trade.

If you can find a doula you click with and who shares your vision, do what you can to hire her, even if your due date is tomorrow. We've all gotten the call, "My due date is in three days." Once I even got a call, "My due date was two days ago." While it's optimal to hire a doula well before your due date, hiring one late in the game is still immensely beneficial.

## Why Invite a Doula?

*If a doula were a drug, it would be unethical not to use one.*
— Klaus, Kennell, and Klaus
*Mothering the Mother*

The following are the potential health benefits of using a doula (see References for Doula Studies):
- 60% reduction in epidural requests
- 40% reduction in Pitocin use
- 50% reduction in Cesarean section
- 25% reduction in labor time
- 30% reduction in additional pain drug use
- Reduced chances of maternal fever and infection
- Reduced incidence of postpartum depression
- Parents have higher regard and increased sensitivity toward babies
- Greater parental satisfaction with the birth
- Decreased risk of postpartum depression
- Increased breast-feeding success

Here are more benefits to the father and mother:

- The doula is trained and knows comfort measures (nurses may or may not).
- The doula is there only for the mother and her partner, no other responsibilities (like monitoring, charting, helping another nurse, health of mother and baby, servicing the machines, etc).
- The doula will help you assert and verbalize your goals and will notify you if there is a deviation from your plans or wishes.
- A doula helps keep the birth atmosphere calm, peaceful, and sacred.
- The doula is familiar with terminology so can help the mother and partner understand what is being said, if caregivers become too technical/medical in their explanations.
- If something does go differently than expected, all the caregivers will be very busy doing what they are supposed to do, and the busier they are the less time they will have for explanations and reassurances. The doula can give a running commentary and still provide physical and emotional support, which may be more important at that moment than it was before.

- A doula allows the partner to participate to his/her comfort levels, without feeling nervous about the aspects he/she may not be so comfortable about.
- There is no change of shift for the doula, while nurses will most likely change at least once during a mom's stay in the labor room.
- The doula is a continuous presence, and as such has a trusting relationship with the mother and partner, thereby creating an atmosphere where the mother feels free to relax and surrender.
- Doulas take turns with the partner doing the harder, more physical parts of labor support, including just offering an extra set of hands and another heart and brain.
- The presence of a doula allows brief breaks and breathers for a partner since someone will always be with the mom

The second-best thing to hiring a doula is to hire an independent midwife (not a hospital CNM) if she isn't already your primary caregiver, that is. Most midwives I know are willing to charge a fee less than their midwifery services for anything from phone consultations to doula services. It's certainly an option worth exploring.

And if neither of those options are available to you, try looking for a La Leche League leader or other moms who have achieved the same kind of birth you are looking to create. They may not be as qualified as a doula or midwife in being your guide through birth, but it's better than going it alone, that's for sure.

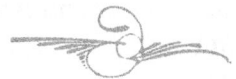

## Exploring Your Birth Beliefs

*Top Ten Myths about Labor and Birth*
*In other words – all these statements are false!*
1. Vaginal exams in late pregnancy are necessary and carry no risks.[25]

2. The best position to push a baby out in is semisitting with legs in stirrups.[26]
3. Wearing monitoring belts continuously throughout labor makes for a healthier outcome.[27]
4. IVs are benign and have no risks.[28]
5. Epidurals always provide the desired pain relief and have no real serious side effects.[29]
6. Waterbirth is very dangerous.[30]
7. Epidural anesthesia and/or Pitocin does not cross the placenta and numb and/or over-stimulate the baby.[31]
8. America has the lowest Cesarean rate in the world.[32]
9. America has the lowest infant death rate in the world.[33]
10. It is dangerous to birth anywhere but the hospital.[34]

Your birth beliefs are actually quite easy to figure out. First, please understand that just because you espouse a belief, that doesn't mean it's true. A belief is a choice. For example, that a baby can be delivered vaginally is not a belief, it's a fact. But to say that a vaginal birth is or isn't healthy for you is a belief. The same could be said of surgical birth.

Your beliefs lead you to your perceptions, your perceptions lead you to your feelings, your feelings impact your decisions, and your decisions determine your outcome and health, which makes up the quality of your life.

So, wouldn't you say that your beliefs are incredibly important? Don't you owe it to yourself and your baby to see that your beliefs are at least based in truth and not in a culture of fear?

If you change your beliefs about yourself, about your false tribal beliefs, and negative perceptions about your present circumstances, then you change your future and your birth and parenting experience and relationships. If you want to change your present and future for the better, you have to adopt truths and beliefs that serve your faith, not your fear.

Now again, review the personal and birth beliefs you wrote down at the beginning of the chapter and honestly answer whether you believe them to be true, possibly true, possibly false, or false. No matter what your beliefs are for any of them, I urge you to go find out if your beliefs are rooted in fact or fear. Research multiple sources for answers.

Be open to your guides and mentors pointing out destructive beliefs that need to be replaced. Ask them to reflect your beliefs back to you. It's okay to identify these destructive beliefs and decide to let them go, then replace them. Write down your new beliefs and keep them with you.

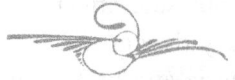

## What Do You Want Your Birth to Look Like?

Go ahead and start by thinking in reverse, and identify what you don't want, then replace those items with the opposite, and plug in visuals to your birth.

If you don't want a Cesarean, tell yourself, "I want a vaginal birth" and see yourself birthing vaginally.

Other affirmations you can use to replace negative mind chatter:

- I want support and autonomy
- I want to be able to easily pay for my dream birth
- I want a caregiver with a philosophy that matches mine
- I want to give birth [at home, in XYZ hospital, in XYZ birth center, in my backyard, you name it]
- I want a waterbirth
- I want a natural birth
- I want a comfortable (i.e., pain-free) birth
- want a healthy baby
- I want a stronger relationship with my partner as a result of this birth
- I want peace

There's a great line in the movie *What about Bob?* that my kids love and repeat back to me when I ask them to be quiet. The dad (Richard Dreyfuss) yells at his son and Bob (Bill Murray), "I want some peace and quiet around here!"

"I'll be quiet," Bob replies.

"I'll be peace," his son says, snickering, while holding up his two fingers in a V.

Truly, if you want peace in your birth—in your life—you really do have to be the embodiment of peace.

> *You must be the change you wish to see in the world.*
> —Mahatma Ghandi

I'm sure there will be people reading this who may go so far as to write me a letter telling me why they can't achieve their peaceful birth experience. In fact, I hope those people do read this book and send me a letter, because it will help them along in their process. But, the list of 'I can't because" could be endless:

- I can't because of my partner
- I can't because of my financial situation
- I can't because of my age
- I can't because I can't find anyone to help me

Believe me, I think I've heard them all. People say they can't ask for help, they can't change their health, they can't change their baby's position, they can't because they'll be disowned or left. Look, it's as simple as this: Just start asking for help and looking for solutions. They are out there.

"But I've had three C-sections, it's too dangerous to birth the way I want to."

"But I am pregnant with twins and can't find anyone to help me with what I want to achieve."

Is it too dangerous? Have you really looked? I mean *dug* for the information?

Is there really no one to help you? Did you know that it is entirely possible and within your realm of influence, to birth twins full term *and* vaginally? All the twin births I've attended have been both full term and vaginal.

And did you know that there are studies out there proving that a VBAC, even after three Cesareans, is safe?[35]

I bet someone is within driving distance who can help you.

"But my husband refuses to agree to what I want to do."

I hate to tell you so bluntly, but he doesn't have to agree. If you stay in faith, peace, understanding and love, the birth will either end up the way you want it anyway, without fighting, or else when it comes time for labor and birth he will be (or will make himself) unavailable.

Love—far and away—is a more powerful force than fear, ego, and anger. You will accomplish more by being loving and understanding without compromising than you will by fighting and pleading your case.

> When my youngest was almost three, I remember thinking back on her birth—a home birth with a wonderful midwife. It was a beautiful, very peaceful and laid-back birth—right up my alley. I realized that day, however, that my husband barely made it to the party. He almost slept through it. My mom woke him up minutes—and I mean less than five minutes before our daughter made her grand entrance into the world.
>
> I'd thought and joked about this before, but this was the first time I really analyzed and digested this fact. It wasn't totally his fault. I sent him to bed, telling him I thought this was the night and that I'd wake him when I needed him. Everything happened pretty fast. I almost waited too long to call my midwife and mom—not wanting to wake them up before it was necessary. They got there only about 40 and 20 minutes before birth.
>
> I could have asked my husband to stay up with me, I could have woken him up before I called the midwife. I realized that morning, three years later, that we were both happier with the way things played out than if he had been there every second of the experience. He was there when it counted and when it mattered most to me, to him, and most especially to our daughter.
>
> I should go back and explain some things. I don't know if my husband is pro-home birth or not. Our first was born in hospital with a midwife—I think he was pretty comfortable with this situation. But with our subsequent kids, I wanted a different experience. He has never jumped on the bandwagon; he is difficult to read and he does not tell all his friends and family what life-changing events our

home births were. Yet he left the choice up to me, even though I believe he would make a different choice.

He went to meet the midwife in her office for the first visit, but never came again—even when we did ultrasounds to see if it was a boy or girl. Because his attitude was the way it was, I've decided I would not want him there. I ended up cherishing the appointments I had with my midwife alone or when my mom, sisters, or best friend were with me. Frankly, it just would not have been the same if he had been there. The same goes for the actual birth. For me, it was easier to be on my own, not worrying about what my husband was thinking—wondering if my midwife would say something he thought was a little weird. I could be myself and enjoy the experience.

Is he a bad husband? Certainly not! He supported me the best way he could given the choices he made. He didn't pressure me to choose something outside my comfort level, and I returned that respect. It might be a weird dynamic, but after years of wondering if we are dysfunctional, I've realized that we naturally let each other remain reasonably comfortable in a situation that could be potentially volatile.

While I honestly think he would still be most comfortable if I gave birth in a hospital, he trusts and respects my instincts. I have not pushed him to be more involved, and I have realized that we can both have a beautiful experience without him being involved in every single step along the way.

Lori, mother of three

While it's maybe your ideal to have a supportive, involved partner for the birth, you have to accept that the only person you can control is you. You can't force him to learn about birth. You can't force him to agree with you. You can only inspire and surrender your perceived control over his mind and heart. Believe that the birth will unfold as peacefully as possible, with or without his emotional or literal support, and trust that the void will be filled.

"But I don't have money for [a doula, home birth, childbirth classes]."

The solution to this is either you trust that the money will appear when needed, you can trade for services, or people can offer their services for free. Everyone has experienced an unexpected increase in money when they needed it for something. Whether it was $5 found in a pocket, a quarter found in the gutter, or a refund check you didn't know was coming, we've all had it happen. If it can happen for $5, why not more than that? If you have a clear intent, a certain amount you desire, and faith that it will show up, more than likely it will.

And personally, I can't count how many times I've traded services and have attended my fair share of pro bono births. I've even taken $5 a week for years until payment is completed! Look, money isn't as much of a barrier as you think it is. Just start looking around, asking, and dreaming.

"But my baby is breech or transverse. No one will work with me."

First of all, examine your options for a breech. What you have been told may not be true. Research and look. Secondly, it is widely accepted, although not scientifically validated, by many birth professionals that the baby's position toward the end of pregnancy is closely tied to the mother's emotional state, and addressing any emotional upsets is in order.

"I want an out-of-hospital birth, but my home isn't suitable and there are no birth centers around me."

Odds are, unless you live in a dangerous environment, your house is fine. I've attended births in mansions and births in trailer homes. Rethink this excuse. Secondly, if your home truly is unsuitable, there are other places to birth, like a hotel. In fact, in Las Vegas there's been plenty of births in the hotel casinos—everywhere from the Bellagio to Circus Circus. You could also seek out a friend's home, or even your midwife's office. Get creative.

> *Two roads diverged in a wood, and I— / I took the one less traveled by, / and that has made all the difference.*
> —Robert Frost

"I can't achieve my peaceful birth because of my health."

That baby is still inside of you, improve your health! Some

changes in diet and lifestyle take effect in as little as 24 hours. I've been a doula at a successful vaginal birth of a paraplegic woman, known of women to change their RH- or GBS+ status, stopped preterm labor on their own, reversed toxemia, and more. You *can* overcome your health obstacles.

While all your excuses seem completely legitimate right now, it's entirely possible that you are lying to yourself. If you believe your lies, then you have no choice, right? And therefore, no responsibility in the outcome. But if you believe that you can rise above your excuses, even just a half step, than there's a way to progress. So, right here, right now, write down all your "I can't because" statements:

_____

_____

_____

_____

_____

_____

_____

_____

_____

_____

_____

These are your excuses and probable falsehoods you tell yourself. Now, ask yourself if there is any possible, infinitesimal way at all to rise above these excuses, even just a bit. Have you even tried to find out if there's a way around them? Or have you just accepted what you've been told? Has anyone else ever found their way around the same excuses you have? If after looking and searching you said no, I would be utterly shocked.

And what if all your reasoning just disappeared? What if, through no work of your own, your health improved, you had a windfall of money, your husband became agreeable, your doctor told you he was fine with whatever you wanted to do, you found new caregivers, your baby turned, what now? Are you scared? Excited? Liberated? Whatever your feeling is, that is your biggest clue behind reaching your peaceful birth.

Act as if all these barriers were gone, and you will start moving toward your peaceful birth. Act as if the universe is handing you a Get-Out-of-Jail-Free card, and all your answers to your "I can't" statements are within your reach, and you will find them.

Focusing on what you do want for your birth really does have astounding effects. The following story, which could have been full of "I can't because" statements is evidence of that.

### The Birth of Zephyr

*I found out I was pregnant with Zephyr right in the middle of multiple crises. My husband was just coming off of a long, life-threatening illness wherein he couldn't work, but he still wasn't completely well and the money was long gone. It took me quite awhile to confirm the pregnancy because I really didn't want to deal with all the loose ends that can come along with pregnancy, but also I had no money for a pregnancy test. I literally had to save up for it. I can't remember taking or reading the test, but what I do remember was being happy and scared. I was so grateful for this baby, but in my head it was the worst timing in the world.*

*Also, frankly, I was worried about people's reactions and judgment. Because it was the worst time, I just didn't want to hear anything negative about it. I really wanted to enjoy it as much as possible. Little did I know that the* timing of the pregnancy was actually perfect. But I wouldn't find that out until the day of the birth.

So, on to the next question, How am I going to have this baby? Not "how" as in, gee how does the baby get from the inside to the outside, but "how" as in no money plus wanting to have another homebirth plus midwife in another city—that how. I contacted Kaye, my friend and one of my midwives, and informed her that I was "in the way" and basically laid out the situation to her to see what her thoughts were. Here's where the answer to this loaded question just got handed to me. It just so happens that Kaye was planning on moving an hour from me around the time of the birth, and oh yeah, don't worry about paying her. The odds of her closing her midwifery practice of 25 years, uprooting her life, and moving closer to me right around due-date time had been slim at best. So I knew that this was another lesson in trusting and surrendering. I was going to be taken care of.

At my first prenatal, we went to her office and I did an ultrasound to narrow down due dates with her, because as always (this was my fifth pregnancy), I don't really have a clue when I conceived. So we determined it could be one of two dates, June 10 or June 18.

I circled Sunday, June 15, as the birth day I wanted. I always loved Sunday births, and it gave us ample time before our moving day, July 1. And it was the happy medium between the two dates, so I thought that was quite reasonable.

The pregnancy progressed uneventfully. All went smoothly and—besides not being able to satisfy my every craving and having to cook every single thing I ate from scratch because I couldn't afford convenience foods or eating out—I really had no complaints.

So fast forward to June 2008. It was the first time I'd ever experienced false labor. It was quite annoying and had my husband in a tizzy a few times. He had been commuting four hours north for his new job since the first of April, which had been a pain, but come June I was used to that, but not used to his nervousness about the birth. He started stressing out that he'd be up north when I went into labor. I told him not to worry about it, it would work out. June 10 came and went with little fanfare.

"C'mon! The baby was supposed to be here by now! Let's go!"

"Wait for the 15th," I'd say.

So Sunday the 15th came and went. I'd lie if I said I wasn't disappointed, but, oh well, I guess the 18th due date was more accurate. We debated whether he should go back up north to work. I told him to just go and I'd call at the slightest twinge (which I didn't, given the false labor stuff).

So, the 16th . . . nuthin.

The 17th . . . nuthin.

The 18th! Due date! Nuthin.

So, he really was getting ants in his pants. We're moving soon, so we were living in a house with a mattress on the ground, blow-up beds, a futon, and one chair and ottoman to nurse in after the baby came. I'm pregnant and playing single mom to four active kids. We have to be gone by July 1, and he's commuting. But I say, "What can we do but just wait and be patient?"

19th . . . nuthin.

20th . . . nuthin.

21st . . . What is the point of waiting for the water to boil anyway? Let's go have some fun. So I piled the kids into the van and went to watch the Shakespearean Festival's Greenshow. I dragged my overdue bum with lawn chairs and a blanket in tow, set up shop, and started the show. I see a few friends.

"Aren't you due?" "Wasn't that baby supposed to be here by now?"

Legitimate questions, since I learned early on to be very vague about due dates. I just gave it up, though.

"Yep, I'm either 11 days or 3 days overdue!"

Ah, those are priceless looks you get when you say that. I'll miss them!

During the Greenshow, I was contracting, but again, I had had many false starts and wasn't really taking anything seriously. Scott had gotten home from up north while we were at the show and when I did get home around 7:45 I was actually in good spirits. But by 8:30 I was still contracting a bit. Huh, I thought.

I knew Kaye had been making runs back and forth to her new home since June 4. I thought maybe I should call her just to see where she was. I hesitantly give her a call, because I didn't want to bug her without just cause.

So, I call.

"Hey, where are you?"

"I am 10 minutes from you."

"Oh! You want to come see if anything's going on with me?"

"Sure!"

Odds of her being 10 minutes from me right when I wanted her? Zero to none. At the time I didn't think much of it, but now I know it was Divine intervention. When she came, I realized she's got two of her boys with her, her daughter, and her son-in-law (who was driving separate). Ah, man, I really didn't want to inconvenience family members too. I told Kaye that I really didn't think I was in labor, but the contractions, even though not so much increasing in frequency or strength, were still going on.

So, she talks me into an exam. I'm 3–4 cm, 100% effaced, and a good +3 station. Well, all fine and good, but that doesn't really mean I'm in labor. I told Kaye to just go home, sorry to bother. But she kind of insisted on staying. I said "Okay, but I'm not guaranteeing anything." She left at 9:00 to tell her family to move on without her, and came back around 9:30ish.

For the next hour and a half, it was kind of more of the same. Maybe a little more intense and closer together, but nothing to get excited about and declare "This is it!" I certainly wouldn't describe it as painful, just interesting. We put the girls to bed about 11:00, and then I noticed things pickup. Still not painful, just more. And then a good contraction came at 11:30.

"Kaye, what do you think about checking me again?"

11:55. I'm something like 5–6 cm and my water broke during the exam. Well, I guess this is it. I decided to run to the bathroom for one last hurrah in there, and had the "contraction of awareness," I guess you could call it. I went from "Maybe this could be it" to, "Ah, crap, oh my gosh, things have to stop now" within three contractions.

I raced back to the front room, took my station on my knees leaning over the futon and let the good times roll. I got maybe 40 seconds between contractions at first, but it quickly went to what felt like only 15 seconds between contractions. Mr. Toad's Wild Ride had begun, keep your hands and feet inside the car at all times, and you aren't getting off until I say so. My neighbor, Ginger, had come at this point, which was a welcome comfort. Everyone but my 3-year-old had come back out of their rooms and we all went on this ride together.

Zephyr was born at 1 a.m., so that means I was in active, hard labor for only an hour. That sounds great to most people, but if you've ever had a quick labor, you know that it is full of its own pros and cons. My fourth birth was a pretty hard birth, but Zephyr's was incredibly hard. His head was big and it took all my strength to get it out. I remember crying after he came out, not because I was overcome by motherly emotion, but because I was so glad to have that head out of me. It was rough.

In my previous labors, they were longer and afforded me some choice spiritual experiences during the actual labor and birth. But Zephyr's was so fast and hard that there was really nothing there. At first I was a bit disappointed that I wasn't afforded the spirituality of the girls' birth, but in reflection, his whole coming into being was a massively spiritual experience.

The next day I woke up with my pretty purple baby (bruised from his speedy entrance) and immediately thought about how I only have one week to recover and finish packing.

Also, because he was so purple for so long, there was a question for that whole week if something was wrong with him. Should we take him to a pediatrician (something

I don't do lightly)? Is there a dangerous heart problem? Why is he soooo purple? Is it really just bruising? Is he going to die? It was hard to get a clear answer. I was tired, had hemorrhoids, nursing like crazy, had four other kids underfoot, was moving to a house I hadn't seen before to a place I didn't know, and had few of my earthly comforts around. It was a trial I don't want to repeat.

I should have been stressing given my lack of proper babymooning. I had had such nice babymoons in the past. But I was reminded of pioneer women birthing on the trail, so I wouldn't feel too sorry for myself. Really, it was fine, just not optimal.

In reflection, the miracles and gifts I was given for his birth were:

Had he been conceived any later, it wouldn't have given me time to recover properly.

Had he been conceived any sooner, Kaye might not have been able to attend me.

Had I not called Kaye when I did, it would have been a massive pain getting her there and she might have missed the birth.

Had Kaye not been the saint she was to attend me for free, well . . . I just don't want to think about what that would have looked like.

Had Scott not left work when he did that day, he may have missed the birth.

Had I not been given multiple distractions postpartum, I may have overreacted to Zephyr's color and intervened unnecessarily.

Had I not surrendered to the timing and wisdom beyond my own, I would have been miserable. And I was done being miserable. I wanted to be happy. And really I was and am so grateful I decided to be in a place of faith rather than fear.

Trust, Surrender, Acceptance, Faith.

Amy, mother of 5

As I pointed out, most people plan their births around money, health, false information, and others' tribal birth values—all of which seem completely valid on the surface. They are allowing a whole lot of distraction to take over their birth experience instead of getting real with themselves. What do you, and therefore your baby, need? What do you want? When you hand your power over to other people and things, that's exactly where your power will end up; in your caregiver's hands, in your lacking bank account, in your lies, in your bad health. When you hand your power over to things and people you don't want to hand them over to, your birth will manifest according to their belief system. Which could lead to a healthy outcome; nonetheless, it's not an experience you will grow from and own.

> The more fear that we live in, the more that we allocate our energy into protection. But you get that energy by taking it away from growth.
> —Bruce Lipton
> *The Wisdom of Your Cells*

You are the one with the last say, you know. Knowing your options and choosing what you actually want is key to getting it. You can have a healthy, peaceful birth of *your* choosing.

During one portion of my childbirth education classes, I lead the couples in a guided imagery exercise. We dim the lights, put on relaxing music, and I tell them to settle in and get comfortable. Setting the mood, like for a date. For some, they stay seated on the sofa, others slouch down in the sofa, and others feel free to grab a pillow and lay down on the floor. Then I have everyone close their eyes and take at least three deep, full breaths. I then have them identify any tension or stressful events of the day and tell them to send them on their way. Just dissolve all their worries. Then I set the stage. I start to paint a picture of an event for them. I describe the weather, time of day, and a sense of calm and happiness within themselves. I proceed to "walk" them through the very first twinges of labor. Then it's on to the intensity a woman begins to feel and finally the releasing of their baby and immediate postpartum.

Reaction to this exercise is varied. I've had couples cry, others hug and kiss, and yet some seem completely unaffected.

The comments from the women or couple who've been moved

by the exercise tend be something like this, "That was incredible! I can't wait to do that!"

Comments from the few unaffected couples go something like this, "I guess that was nice, but I couldn't get into it. I couldn't put myself there."

While the majority of those unaffected couples go on to have wonderful births, they tend to have one thing in common after this exercise. Either they are still undecided about their birth plans or they are caught up in making "the right" decisions. Usually these people live their lives in the same fashion. They are afraid to make a move in case they choose incorrectly. The irony here is that their pregnancy and birth will progress whether they make decisions or not and will take on a life of its own unless they take the wheel and direct it themselves. To me, being caught up in being right, and putting off decision making *is* making a decision and it's the wrong one.

Go ahead and try to mentally walk yourself through the labor and birth of your dreams. Can you place yourself, your mind, your wishes in the scenarios of your peaceful birth? You know what you want, the question is can you admit it, own it, and see it in your mind's eye?

My good friend and colleague Jonelle and I use to joke how we could write an entire book on all the "what if" questions our students and clients presented us. All these what if's are more or less based on your limiting beliefs about yourself and tribal beliefs you've been handed, not birth itself. It would be nice to say at this point in the book, "Okay, I've completed the hardest steps to achieving my peaceful birth, there's nothing left to do but just sit back and wait." But there's all those inconvenient what if's lurking inside you and waiting to manifest. Let me elaborate on this point.

I grew up the youngest of six children with a great stay-at-home mom and hard-working father. We went out to eat at a sit-down restaurant as a family six times a year, to celebrate each of our birthdays. I don't remember ever ordering for myself. I think my dad may have ordered for all of us, but at any rate, I remember always being aware that price was important. The most bang for the buck, the better. But it didn't matter to me. I loved going out to eat those six times a year—or less, as my siblings left home to start their own families. I just enjoyed being out with my family, trying something new and not having to make anything or clean up.

In no way am I criticizing or complaining about this aspect of my upbringing, that price was important. In fact, there were some good lessons in it. Having a large family of my own now, I totally get where my parents were coming from in this approach to eating out.

Fast forward to my second date with my future husband. We went to a mid-priced national restaurant chain to eat dinner. I had never really been one for dating, so I still had very limited experience in being taken out to dinner. Up until this point I had chosen boyfriends who spent very little money on me. In fact, they sometimes expected me to pay for them because of their meager earnings, which always rubbed me the wrong way, especially when I wasn't warned they were expecting me to pay for a date they asked me on. Duh.

So, there we were, seated at the booth. I opened the menu, and being sort of new to eating out, got a bit overwhelmed and my knee-jerk reaction was to choose the cheapest thing on the entrée list. Shoot, I was even considering getting just an appetizer for dinner based on price. Anyway, I choose a quesadilla, priced at $7.19. My future husband took a little while to decide, so I had some time to actually look at all the other menu choices. I spied something that I really wanted—a chicken Caesar salad. I had never had one, but had always heard how good they were. But it was $7.99.

My date asked me what I was getting. I said, "Either the quesadilla or Caesar salad." I looked up at him to test his reaction. Almost as if I was seeking his approval for the meal he was paying for. He really had no reaction, just a kind of "huh, okay, whatever" body language. Then I said, "Oh, I'll just get the quesadilla, I guess."

He picked up on my reluctance, "Do you want the salad?"

"Well, yeah, but it's more expensive and I'll be just as happy with the quesadilla."

"Get the salad if you want that. Eighty cents isn't going to kill me. In fact, get the steak if you want to. Then we'll get dessert, too," he said smiling.

"Where's the steak on the menu?" I said.

I didn't even know the place offered steak, because all I had done was scan the prices, paused at the lower priced ones, and considered those. Ah, I found it. The steak was $13.99?! That's a 1 with a 3 and 99 after the decimal. I don't think so. I couldn't do that. What would he think of me? What if he thought I was greedy? What if he thought I was ungrateful? What if he thought I was trying to take advantage of his paying for the meal? What if, what if, what if.

I didn't even realize I was placing this limit on myself. And I certainly didn't see that there might be a problem with placing that limit on myself until it was pointed out to me. What I didn't understand was the implications of the reverse of all those what ifs What would he think of me if I only limited myself to the cheapest thing on the menu? What if he thought I was stingy? What if he thought I didn't think much of myself? What if he thought I thought he was a cheapy cheapo?

My husband became a good mentor in some aspects of money for me. And that's certainly what most, if not all, parents-to-be need. You need a birth guide to illuminate your choices and strengths and remind you that you have no limits. To address your what ifs that might come up after you've made your decisions and help put them aside. And definitely don't let 80 cents (something minor and inconsequential in the long run) keep you from realizing your dream birth.

By the way, I ordered the salad, and frequently order it nowadays

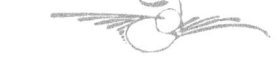

## Claiming the Territory

Don't expect people to be psychic. You have to communicate, most of the time in writing, what you want. You have to believe that what you want is attainable and feel the loving energy from it. Some people call this a birth plan. Over the years, my idea of an effective birth plan has morphed significantly.

When I was pregnant with my first, I had a three-page—yes, *three*—birth plan. It not only listed what I wanted, but the tone of it assumed the worst of the staff:

> "I don't want an unnecessary Cesarean."
> "No continuous electronic fetal monitoring."
> "No separation."

No this, no that. The fact that those nurses just smiled and nodded when I handed it to them, I am grateful for that. Reading it now, any nurse would have been justified in being insulted by it. It breaks my heart to know the condescension and eye-rolling that some moms-to-be with birth plans like my first one get. And in some regards, it's understandable. Not right, but understandable. An assumptive negative birth plan is just plain rude. Maybe not intentionally rude, but your fear on the paper translates into the nurses feeling like you assume they are out to get you.

Even just slightly less annoying are those website-generated, scripted, impersonal birth plans. Just click your preference and print. So easy, right? More like, so empty. How can anyone take you seriously when such little thought, effort, and heart is put into shaping the most significant event of your life?

> A goal casually set and lightly taken will be freely abandoned at the first obstacle.
>
> —Zig Ziglar

All the professionals on your birth team are going to pick up on the vibe of your birth plan. The specific words, length, or detail of the birth plan really is inconsequential. It's your passion and desire, or lack of it, that leaps off the page and engages people to support you.

When I took my first doula client, I had a pretty concrete idea of what a natural hospital birth plan should look like. It should look like mine did, right? When she handed me her birth plan, I was confused.

*Dear Doctor _____ and Hospital Staff,*

*We are happy to be delivering with you. We chose you because we are confident you can help us achieve our dream of a natural birth. Please assist us by giving us suggestions and reassurance as we head toward our goal. Our top three aims are that I am able to move freely, hold the baby right after I deliver, and keep the environment peaceful.*

*Sincerely,*
*Suzanne*

Now, if you were a nurse or doctor, wouldn't you rather get something like that than my "no, no, no" birth plan? You do not have to detail out every little thing in your birth plan; the overall energy of it will say that for you. I'd be much more willing to support someone with the attitude my client took than someone expecting a fight, like I did.

I quickly learned that the kind of birth plan that my first client wrote is the most effective. Even more effective is when the client hands the nurses donuts, cookies, or a gift with the birth plan. Those nurses work hard, long, and sometimes thankless hours. It makes a difference for them, and you, when you are thoughtful and charitable toward them. A little bit of honey can go a long way. What puts the cherry on top of it is if you and/or your doula send a thank-you letter, pointing the nurses out by name. Sometimes I do this even before the birth to visualize being effective in helping my client achieve the birth she wants, leaving space for the names and filling them in afterward.

I remember the birth of one of my oldest friend's baby. She had delivered twice before with the practice she hired for this third birth, and also at the same hospital. Both times the births went well, with only minor glitches. She didn't have any reason to anticipate that this third birth wouldn't go the same way. I had attended those two other births and, given the nature of our friendship, our professional relationship was informal, to say the least. With her and her husband's permission, I invited Jonelle to come to this birth with me, just to enhance the birth experience.

When we got to the hospital, my friend was well established in active labor and the nurse was trying to talk her into accepting an IV, something she had avoided with no problems in her previous births. This poor, greenie nurse tried every excuse under the sun to convince my laboring friend to accept the IV, to no avail. Finally, the nurse brought in backup - the head nurse. Tensions started to rise between the nurses and my friend and her husband. The nurses convinced them that if my friend didn't have a temperature then they were fine with her laboring without an IV, and they agreed, certain that there would be no problem and the matter could be put to rest. Her temperature was .2 degrees above normal. 98.8 degrees instead of 98.6. That's all the nurses needed to pressure them further. I don't know, she was working hard at 6 cm; I thought that .2

degrees above normal was totally reasonable!

My friend's husband threatened to leave. They'd call a midwife and have a home birth. Well, you could tell that this was not something the nurses had ever handled before. They backed off and both parties "compromised" (there's that word again) on doing a hep lock instead of an IV. The rest of the birth went quickly and smoothly, and the OB on call, who my friends had actually never met before, turned out to be really great and accommodating, going so far as to suggest to my friend's husband catch the baby, which he did.

As much as Jonelle and I tried to bridge gaps and calm waters, we left knowing those nurses weren't happy with that birth. We had always written thank-you letters to the attending staff for the births we went to, but we knew we had to get this one out ASAP.

Our thank-you letter praised them and their patience and professionalism. We acknowledged that the situation wasn't ideal but thanked them by name for the care they gave and that they ultimately set things aside to give our friend a good birth experience.

Two months later Jonelle attended a birth at that same hospital. I got a call at 11 p.m.

"You aren't going to believe what I'm standing in front of," she said.

"What? Where are you?"

"I am standing in front of our thank-you letters."

"Huh?"

"Kim's birth. That new redhead nurse . . ."

"Are you serious?"

"Like a heart attack."

"Spill it."

"So I come in with my client and lo and behold, it's redhead nurse at check-in. I was a little hesitant, but her face lit up when she saw me. She totally welcomed us, got us settled in, and then thanked me for our letters. She said that her supervisor was so impressed with her that she would leave such a great impression."

"Shut up!"

"I swear it. So then she tells me that if there is anything I need, just ask. She told me to feel free to use the nurses' lounge to get ice or whatnot. So I do, and this is what I find. Our letters."

"Wow. That is awesome!"

"Okay, I've gotta get back to the birth."

Can you imagine her reception of Jonelle and her client if we hadn't written those letters? Handwritten gratitude and love go a long way.

Think back to when I described how I walk my childbirth education students through a birth in their minds. To be perfectly honest with you, it's a waste of time to do this visualization if the students aren't willing to put themselves in the middle of the visualization. They need to smell it, hear it, touch it, and feel it as best they can. Then is when it becomes truly transformative and effective. Why? How? Scientists have located the seat of emotions through imaging technology, and the activity in the brain, and we know that the strength and number of neural connections associated with a thought or behavior are increased when you're in a highly emotional state.

The neuron connections are also stronger, longer lasting and it takes longer to lose a neural connection when it was formed with great emotion.[36]

So, if you've researched your options, gotten proper support, stepped into a consistent way of being peaceful, then you are ready to create the details of your birth. Go ahead and write out your birth experience from beginning to end:

_____

_____

_____

_____

_____

_____

_____

_____

Now, take that and add more detail, from even before the first twinge of change to an hour or two postpartum. What's the weather like? Time of day? Any pleasing scents? Sounds? Food or drink you'd like? Length of time? Level of comfort? Labor positions? Birth positions? Home? Birth Center? Hospital? What are you wearing?

The sky's the limit. There are no barriers in your brain, and no harm in creating what you want, not what you think you have to do, mentally and emotionally. Now, write it again, with much more detail, in the past tense as if it's already happened:

_____

_____

_____

_____

_____

_____

_____

_____

_____

_____

_____

_____

_____

_____

_____

Read, visualize, feel, smell every little detail of this experience at least once every day for a minimum of 28 days. Why 28? Most processes within the human body happen in 28 days. For instance, it takes 28 days to replace the cells of a human being's epidermis completely. Women's menstrual cycle is 28 days, the linings of the stomach and intestines are new every 28 days. By visualizing with intense emotion your ideal birth for 28 days, it is more likely that it will become part of your cell memory and easier for you to achieve.[37] If you don't have 28 days left in your pregnancy, do it anyway because it can't hurt. If you have more than 28 days, then great! New research has shown that 66 is the average number of days it takes to form habits. In the study, they looked at how long it took people to reach a limit of self-reported automaticity for performing a new behavior (that is, performing an action automatically), and the average time was 66 days. To create a habit you need to repeat the behavior in the same situation. It is important that something about the setting where you perform the behavior is consistent so that it can cue the behavior. This may be one reason why home birthers are on average more successful in achieving their intended outcome, because their brains are already habituated to relax and surrender in their environment. On that same note, if you are not having a home birth, doing something to create a setting cue, such as wearing the same clothes during the visualization as you are during the birth, might increase your odds of this exercise being effective.[38]

This exercise can take two minutes or an hour, but the more detail and emotion you add and feel, the better it works. I recommend it before going to sleep at night so the peaceful, powerful energy lingers in your subconscious throughout the night. In fact, if you can record your script and listen to it on a loop through the night, even better. Live, eat, feel, breathe, dream, and pray your experience as if it's already happened so you can more easily manifest it.

You may be questioning the validity of my 28-day walk with your dream birth, so let me elaborate a bit further.

In yoga there is a concept called *samskaras*—patterns in the consciousness.

The way you stand, the way you react to certain smells, the way you breathe, it's all a result of your consciousness. But you usually think about patterning when something you do, such as unconsciously biting your nails or eating without thinking, is driving you nuts and you can't figure out how to stop your behavior.

It's the job of your brain to follow patterns. Your brain neurons *like* doing familiar things.

Every time you repeat a familiar action your neural pathways are actually *strengthened*. So every time you react emotionally in a similar way to someone or something, that neural pathway becomes deeper and more easily traveled by your neurons.

You can picture those neurons pretty easily if you think about water traveling down the side of a hill. The water from a rainstorm doesn't just go any which way. The water finds squiggly little grooves and stick to it. And so it is in your brain, for now.

I've emphasized a lot in this book changing your thought patterns, and it's for this reason. If you have created nueral pathways that aren't productive, you need to change them. The same quality of the brain that made it so easy for your old patterns to form is exactly what's going to help you make new ones.

The brain takes to new things really well, as long as you throw repetition into the mix. In brain science terms it's called neuroplasticity. If you create *new* grooves and pathways, the existing ones will heal up and disappear if left on their own.

Those brain grooves are literal applications of *samskaras*. The easiest way to change your *samskaras* is with practice, love, and patience. Over and over again.

Working on your samskaras gives you freedom, choice, and power, all essential elements to achieving your peaceful birth.[39]

> Don't judge each day by the harvest
> you reap, but by the seeds you plant.
> —Robert Louis Stevenson

Very rarely is it that by the last night of my childbirth class series, or last doula prenatal, that a woman or couple still doesn't know what steps they need to take in order to achieve their peaceful birth. When this happens, I know they haven't been real with themselves. They are letting their fears and self-doubts make their decisions and shape their experiences.

If, after you've done the work put forth in this book, you still don't know what you should do to get what you want in birth, you are fooling yourself. I don't mean to be harsh, but it's the truth. In fact, you probably know what you need to do, without having to read any further. Right under your excuses and fears are your desires. Do yourself a favor, and say it out loud right now. Simply state what you want, in spite of your fears and tribal members.

The only downside to doing this is that you have to take responsibility and own your desires. This is an empowering, defining moment. From here on out, with unconscious and some conscious effort you will start moving in the direction of your peaceful birth, or you will have to continue to grapple and find excuses for why you can't. Either direction might involve you being uncomfortable. Do you think you can stay safe when you're continuing to lie to yourself and repeating the mantra, "I don't know what I want"? This is a dangerous way to live, especially in terms of your birth choices. Liberate yourself by making your choices now.

It's easy to underestimate how difficult it is for someone to become curious. For seven, ten, or even fifteen years of school, you are required not to be curious. Over and over again, the curious are punished.

I don't think it's a matter of saying a magic word; boom! and then suddenly something happens and you're curious. It's more about a . . . process where you start finding your voice, and finally you begin to realize that the safest thing you can do feels risky and the riskiest thing you can do is play it safe.

Once recognized, the quiet yet persistent voice of curiosity doesn't go away. Ever. And perhaps it's such curiosity that will lead us to distinguish our own greatness from the mediocrity that stares us in the face.[40]

Brian Tracy, a self-help guru, conducted a study on goal setting and found that people who simply wrote down their desires and put the list away discovered that a year later 80 percent of what they wrote manifested. So, it's important to write your birth wishes down. Use this space for them:

_____

_____

_____

_____

_____

_____

_____

_____

_____

_____

_____

_____

_____

_____

_____

_____

Did you write down a lot of wishes? As you were writing, how did you feel? Some women even feel embarrassed to admit what they truly want, almost as if they don't deserve it. Or that by acting on their desires they would alienate others and make them feel bad because they felt good.

I was watching the movie *The Color Purple* last night for the first time. In it, Whoopi Goldberg's character, Miss Celie, couldn't bring herself to smile without covering her mouth. She was ashamed to even smile. She was an abused woman who had gone through much hardship and didn't even know how to feel joy anymore.

If this is you, if you are afraid to move forward in the direction of your dreams because of feeling unworthy or guilty, then you have let your tribe do a great job of controlling you. Your poppy has been cut.

Or, as you were writing, did you get a feeling of superiority? That, if you had a birth experience that no one else had, that you will be "better than them," or "prove them wrong"? This is also ego, and is also not conducive to a peaceful birth.

But if, as you were writing, you had thoughts and hopes of everyone, everywhere experiencing such an awesome experience and/or felt an overwhelming sense of love and strength, then you are at one and in tune with that peaceful spirit. You are much more likely to attract and achieve your peaceful birth.

A peaceful birth, independent of the mode or outcome, is much bigger and more powerful than our doubts, fears, and egos. It can surpass everything you imagined. The trick is to humbly ask for what we want without feeling guilt, shame, fear, dominance, or superiority. Be open to your wishes being met in glorious, unexpected ways.

This inner yearning to birth peacefully and powerfully is universal and has come to you from a place bigger than yourself. Now sincerely, unapologetically, and decidedly heed those gut feelings and write down how you really want your birth to unfold:

_____

_____

_____

_____

Okay, now can you stretch your dreams even further? Maybe you wrote down, "I want a healthy baby," which is fine. But what is even better than that? "I want a vibrant, alert, calm, healthy baby." The goal here is to make improvement on your honest desires. So take what you just wrote, and see if you can make your wishes even more spectacular:

_____

_____

_____

_____

_____

_____

_____

_____

_____

_____

_____

_____

_____

Now, close your eyes and think of everything you just wrote. What jumps out at you first? What is illuminated? If it was more than one thing, that is fine. Meditate on your excitement and energy surrounding that wish or wishes, and now write it down in the most powerful statement that you can:

_____

_____

_____

_____

_____

_____

_____

Wasn't that awesome?!
Are you afraid to commit because there is no guarantee? Write it down, yes or no:

_____

What is the guarantee if you *don't* commit?
That's right. You are guaranteed that *none* of your wishes get met if you don't commit to something you want. If your birth plans require a guaranteed good outcome before you can commit to them, you will neither have a commitment to the plans, nor success in them.
There is another side to this coin, though. No matter what you do, you are committing to something. Whether you decide to own

your birth and shape it into what you are drawn to, or you choose to let others shape your birth for you, you are committing to something. I will guarantee you this: if you claim your territory and shape your birth, you will be happier than if you let others do it for you, even if your birth goes in an unplanned direction. And if you do let others shape your birth for you, there will be a degree of disappointment in yourself and your birth experience, even if you have a healthy birth.

In reality, you are risking more in a very literal and figurative sense by handing the decision making power over to someone else.

To end this section, take the last wish you elaborated on and add the phrase, "Or something greater than I can dream." This allows us to let go of our control and surrender. If you insist on a waterbirth but go on to have a land birth, you will be disappointed. But what if that land birth could have been more fulfilling and easier than the waterbirth could have been? Let go of your control and ego.

I had an acquaintance that, for her third birth, had the baby in the car on the way to the hospital. I had heard this story secondhand, and when I met her for the first time, two weeks after giving birth, I gave her what I considered a compliment. "Oh, that is fantastic! Don't you feel like you can do anything now?" Well, apparently, she didn't. Even though the birth went smoothly and she and the baby were in great health, she was very disturbed by the experience and I could tell that no one had said anything positive to her about it. Not that she could have done anything differently in terms of the physical events, but it was a prime example of how even when a birth goes well, if you aren't willing to surrender, accept, and dream about your birth you will not be happy with it.

This process of surrendering and letting go, as you will see, is an essential element to achieving a peaceful birth. The irony here is that to attain your dream birth you have to desire it without demanding it. We will explore this more in depth later, but for now, add that last bit – 'or something greater' - to your statement.

_____

_____

_____

Look at your statement now. Examine it. Be certain that there is only positive language in there. Nothing like, "I don't want a Cesarean." Tweak it if you need to and make sure every ounce of you feels happy, strong, and positive about your statement.

Now, write it on three cards.

Keep one with you in your wallet or purse. Put the other two cards in places you will see them often. It can be your car, workspace, or pantry. For me, this would be the refrigerator and bathroom (Can you tell what I'm doing all the time? But really, what pregnant woman isn't in either of those two places all the time?). Just by seeing the card, and not even reading it, you are triggering your memory, thinking of it, reinforcing your new neural pathways and pulling yourself toward your goal.

Now for the really good part. Just surrender. Let go and relax. Unseen forces are working on your behalf, moving in the direction of your dreams. Just as your uterus has unseen power and life within it before you even conceived, so do your wishes. And just as you've nurtured, fed, and grown your baby with little effort on your part, the rest of this book will help you nurture and grow your dreams. From here on out, until delivery day, the hardest part of manifesting your peaceful birth may be over.

> The greatest achievements were at first
> and for a time dreams. The oak sleeps
> in the acorn.
>
> James Allen

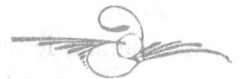

## Of Blessingways and Babymoons

Before I leave you, I want to give you some icing, and decoration, and special effects for this peaceful birthing cake you now have. With my first two babies, I didn't have the opportunity to have the typical baby shower, and maybe it was just as well. Ladies, some I knew well, others I didn't, sitting around, eating cheese and crackers and thick frosted cake from the grocery store. Playing the typical baby shower games—the safety pin one where if you say the word baby or cross your legs and whoever catches you gets your pin. Or the Guess the Melted Candy Bar in the Diaper game. Oh, and there's that one where you have to taste the jar of unlabeled baby food and guess what it is.

Then the gift opening: baby clothes, bottles, pacifiers, and maybe a stroller. It just wasn't me. While that's great for some people, I crave something more meaningful, more intimate, more celebratory. The third time around, like with my first two babies, I wanted to soak up what it really meant to be pregnant, to give birth, to become a mother and family, to feel the real support of my loved ones.

So I asked Jonelle to give me a blessingway.

The story of the creation of the Navajo people and their emergence onto their sacred homeland is recounted in a ceremony known as the blessingway, which is the foundation of the Navajo way of life. A blessingway focuses on the story of Changing Woman, who is the inner form of the Earth through its seasonal transformations. She is the major deity for the Navajo.

The Navajo are instructed that in the beginning, First Man and First Woman emerged onto this world near Huerfano Mountain in New Mexico. One day, First Man found a baby on a nearby mountain. The baby matured in four days and became Changing Woman. Changing Woman created the four original Navajo clans from her body. Her sons rid the land between the four sacred mountains of dangerous monsters and made it safe for the clans to inhabit. The blessingway recounts in detail the instructions Changing Woman gave to the Navajo people she created. These teachings concern history and major religious practices, such as a girl's puberty rite and the consecration of a family's hogan. When performed in its entirety, the blessingway is a two-day ceremony whose purpose is to obtain peace, harmony, protection, and to help realize the goal of a long happy life.

In our culture there are so few ways to honor the mother to be. We make an attempt during baby showers, but for the most part this turns into a simple showering of gifts for the baby and does nothing for the mother in terms of the rite of passage she is about to go through. This sacred time in the mother's life deserves more than gifts of car seats and baby wipes.

While baby showers can be more commercial in focus, the

blessingway serves up a refreshingly sharp contrast. There's no booty of pink and blue gifts. The blessingway is about the woman we know best—our friend and sister, the mother-to-be.

And while society seems eager to chuck aside the mother in favor of holding a cherubic, gurgling baby, a blessingway provides the mother with memories of a true show of support from her loved ones. And that lasts much longer than those newborn sleepers.

Take into account that this is to be an extra-meaningful celebration honoring the woman entering into motherhood and/or welcoming a new life, not necessarily a party for the baby.

*Attendees:* Keep it small, between 6 and 15 guests. Don't invite anyone out of mere courtesy, but make sure the guests are people who really mean something to you and who contribute positively to either your birthing, life, or parenting experiences and who are supportive of your philosophies. These people often include your mother, sisters, or other close female relatives, best friends, midwife, and/or doula. People you would feel free to share your deepest thoughts and cry with. This isn't the time to invite Aunt Edna, whom you only see at funerals, weddings, and the like.

*Location:* Preferably at one of the guest's home, or your own, that has a calm, peaceful, and relaxed feel about it. If this is not an option, a park or some other serene setting can work.

*Atmosphere:* Something akin to a candlelight dinner. Consider playing relaxing music or the honoree's favorite album. Also diffusing essential oils can immediately trigger a wonderful response by the guests and leave them with a sensory memory of the occasion. Turn off all the phones.

*Food:* Typically a blessingway consists of food with some meaning behind it. For instance, you can request that each guest brings a dish that reminds her of her mother or comfort food. Or you can have everyone bring a dish that represents the mother's favorite food groups. For example, if the mother's favorite food is chocolate, have everyone bring a chocolate treat. The point being that it is something homemade and from the heart.

*Blessingway Rituals:* Make sure that whatever you do at a blessingway serves to strengthen and uplift the mother-to-be. Some women are very open to suggestions, others like to do something a little more mainstream, such as a day at the spa or going to a paint-your-own-pottery place. Be open to customizing activities to suit the mother's definition of being uplifted. Consider one of the following:

Request that each guest bring a special bead that reminds them of the mother to be to string on a necklace or bracelet for the mother to wear until and through labor. A nice way to approach this ritual is by sitting in a circle and passing the cord, each guest adding a bead or beads for each number of children they have, then the mother can add a final bead after the birth to represent her own child. The necklace or bracelet symbolizes the strength of our shared experiences as mothers and women.

Similarly, a ball of beautiful string (hemp is durable and works well) is used to connect each woman's wrist to one another's in the circle—a web of womanhood. When the cord connects all of you, explain that this unites you all as sisters and represents the circle of sisters and the circle of life. Then you cut the cord, leaving enough length to tie the ends into a bracelet. Explain that though it appears we were then separate, the bracelet reminded us as women, we were all cut from the same ball of yarn. You may suggest that the women wear the bracelet until the birth as a reminder of the strength a group of women can hold for a birthing mother.

Candle making or giving candles as a party favor is great to include. The reason being is that all the guests will be asked to light the candle when they are notified that the mother is in labor and will leave it lit until the baby arrives.

Smudging is taken from the Navajo origins of the blessingway and is for if the blessingway is taking place in the honoree's home. A bundle of dried sage is often lit, then the flame burned out and the sage is allowed to slowly burn down. This is to symbolize a cleansing of the woman's home, either for a home birth or for the arrival home from the birthplace, purifying of her soul and blessing for the birth and baby.

Belly casting is another ritual that can be fun. Either have the guests cast the mother's belly and chest, or have the cast already done and ready for the guests to paint or decorate. Another belly activity is to henna the mother's belly. Some themes to consider for henna painting and cast decorating:

    Personal Heritage
    Celestial

Nature
Animals
Fairies
Abstract art
Symbolic

Some mediums to consider:

Decoupage
Murals
Mosaics
Dried flowers
Baby heirlooms/keepsakes
Watercolor/tie-dye

Foot washing symbolizes readiness for a journey or new beginning, and hand washing will clean away fears. The feet or hands should be dried and can be smoothed and massaged with cornmeal, or with oils. The midwife or grandmother-to-be is usually the one to honor the mother with these aspects, but it can provide a wonderful time for guests to bestow quiet words of love and encouragement.

Hair brushing and braiding is another way to nurture and pamper the mother. If there is a brush that is, for example, an heirloom, this can act as a way to connect the mother to her female ancestors. Adorning her hair with flowers can also help connect her to Mother Earth.

Song is such a wonderful way to invite a loving spirit. Many women like to have each guest sing a lullaby their mother used to sing or one they have used with their own children. If all the guests are familiar with one particular song, say a lullaby, spiritual or hymn, this can also be sung together as a group.

Send away your troubles and fears by having guests voice them, write them on paper, and then burn them from a bowl and sending them away.

Storytelling of each woman's personal birth stories can be inspiring, but beware if you think horror stories will be passed around. Remember you are strengthening and uplifting the mother! Or listen to stories of how each guest knows the mother or inspirational stories of each guest's relationship to the mother—how they met her, what drew them to her, why she is important to them. This can be done during the hair brushing or foot washing or during candle lighting. This can also take the form of poetry reading or reciting an inspirational story or fable, and either read just one or invite guests to bring a poem or story of their own to read.

Quilting is probably one of the oldest forms of female rituals. It's very meaningful to ask in the invitation for each guest to bring a customized quilt square that tells of a certain quality the mother possesses. Either assemble the quilt at the blessingway, or assign a friend to complete the quilt and present it to the mother and baby after the birth. This will become an heirloom that tells a story about the mother.

A keepsake journal can be passed around during the foot washing or hair brushing for the guests to write down inspirational thoughts or poems. After the birth the mother can write of the baby's birth story.

Compile a "nurture basket." In the invitation, instead of baby gifts, instruct the guests to bring a gift that would uplift, inspire, or nurture the mother. This can be a gift certificate for a massage or restaurant, bath goodies, books or journals, framed quotes, drawings or photos, luxurious robes or pajamas, teas or chocolates, "gift certificates" for postpartum help and meals, etc.

Be respectful of the mother's religious preference, if any. If all the guests are of the same religious background, these aspects should be incorporated into the blessingway.

My own blessingway and ones I have given for other friends have been very powerful, uplifting events. Everyone loves them. Now doesn't that sound better than thick frosted cake and being given a package of diapers?

## Babymooning

Now on to your babymoon. Everyone expects a newly married couple to take some time to themselves after the wedding. It's widely recognized that they need to be given some space so that they can become comfortable in their new roles as husband and wife (to say nothing of beginning to recover from the sheer insanity of those stress-filled weeks leading up to the wedding). But when couples who've just had a baby ask to be given a few days to themselves before the visitors start arriving in droves, they're sometimes made to feel as if they're being unreasonably selfish in depriving other people of the chance to sneak a peek at the new arrival.

> In the sheltered simplicity of the first days after a baby is born, one sees again the magical sense of two people existing only for each other.
> —Anne Morrow Lindbergh

*Babymooning,* a phrase dubbed by renowned childbirth educator Sheila Kitzinger, is where the family takes time alone during a baby's first few days of life. Not only do new mothers need to physically recover from the rigors of giving birth and adjust to the hormonal changes that are triggered as they move from a pregnant to a nonpregnant state, but both parents also need a chance to regain their bearings and get used to the fact that from this point forward they're going to be someone's mom or dad.

It's not like we Westerners invented babymooning at all. Most cultures recognize the need for this time after the birth in order to ensure the baby's survival and to help the family thrive. One tribe in Brazil, for example, gives the mother and baby a month of seclusion. And in India, it's traditional for new mothers to focus solely on meeting the new baby's needs during the first 22 days after the birth. These cultures have long known what we're just now discovering: our bodies and relationships need alone time after a birth. Also, it's only natural to want to drink in everything about your new baby—the softness of her skin, the vulnerability of her cry, the irresistible smell of the top of her head, and those soulful stares that tell you that there's a lot more going on inside her head than you might otherwise have suspected.

All your senses are heightened after birth in order to forge a strong bond to your baby and become acutely aware of what you need in order to stay mentally, emotionally and physically healthy. A babymoon is in order.

> *My sense of smell, taste, and even feeling textures in my mouth and with my fingertips were so enhanced. If something smelled good, it smelled really good. If something tasted bad, I couldn't eat it for weeks after the initial taste. And feeling my baby's skin was like heaven. My hearing was especially affected. What was once the typical volume on the TV was suddenly too loud. I couldn't stand to watch violent movies or anything with a fight in it. And even the thought of listening to semi-harsh music got me stressed out.*
>
> —Penelope, Mother of three, one week after birth

Nature made this heightened state a universal constant for every woman. It's how we bond to our babies and make them and ourselves and families strong.

> *Because I was feeling so good, I made the mistake of going to the store two days after giving birth. What seemed like a normal shopping experience to others ended up being very stressful for me. I felt like everyone was staring at and judging me. I felt so exposed and vulnerable to everyone. Luckily no one came up to me and wanted to touch and ask about the baby. If they had, I might have run out of there.*
>
> Laura, mother of two

Don't make the mistake of assuming that you don't need a babymoon if this is your second or subsequent baby. Babymoons aren't just for first-time parents. In fact, having a babymoon is even more important after your first. Your life and routines seem to get going again all too soon and people aren't as thoughtful because they assume you know more what you're doing and don't need the help as much.

Yes, relatives and friends are well meaning, and even I have been guilty of wanting to pounce on my nieces' and nephews' new bundle, but having visitors all day and night during your first days and week after the birth is just a setup for exhaustion, postpartum depression, and malnourishment of the mother and baby. It can be overwhelming and inhibiting to establishing a strong breast-feeding relationship, and a distraction to taking care of yourself and baby.

Talk to your partner about your plans for the babymoon. It's important to be upfront about your expectations so that there won't be any crossed wires or hurt feelings down the road. Just like it is important to upfront and honest about your partner's level of involvement during labor and birth, so it is important to be realistic and honest with regard to your partner's involvement: while you might want him to participate wholeheartedly in the babymoon experience, you have to be prepared if he isn't willing or able to hang out with you and the baby 24 hours a day. Forcing the issue will only lead to stress and conflict at the time in your life when you most need to feel in sync with your partner. Molly, a 36-year-old mother of three is still dealing with the fallout of her babymoon three years later:

> *I really wanted a babymoon. I had fantasies of my family and I spending hours lying around and falling in love with the baby. My husband I agreed that he would do the dishes, laundry, make the meals, and take care of our daughters during his time off, about five days. Well, I felt great after the birth, a little too great, and my husband took that as a signal that he could do some yard work, make some work phone calls, and spend time on the computer. He would spend about half the day doing things other than caring for me and the family. That left me feeling abandoned and taken advantage of. I ended up having to do the dishes and folding loads of laundry.*

How you spend your time immediately following birth you can never get back and it will be etched in your memory. Whether it's good or bad is a matter of planning. Just like you will always remember your wedding day, your honeymoon, and the day you birthed your baby, you will always remember your babymoon.

Communicate your wishes to friends and family. Once you and your partner have agreed about how you intend to handle your babymoon, be sure to get the word out to friends and family members. You'll find that people will be more accepting of your need for privacy during the early days if they are prepped and you reassure them that there will be ample opportunities for visiting down the road. Another way to handle this situation is to let the eager beavers in the crowd pay a quick visit shortly after the birth: with any luck, they'll back off a little once they've had the chance to check out the baby. But there is still caution with this.

> *My next baby, I'm not going to tell anyone I had her for at least a week. Even well-meaning phone calls and help drained me. I don't really care if they think I'm dead. I regret devoting energy to anyone other than my baby and husband. It's more important to preserve that time with my family.*
> —Stacie, mother of one

How much time for a babymoon? That's going to vary, but plan on at least a week. Some women take the end of their lochia flow as a signal that their body is ready to resume normalcy. For some mothers, especially those who had worked outside the home, they can feel like they have cabin fever, but resisting the urges to go out and do something pays off in the end. That's not to say that a leisurely walk isn't in order, but certainly don't resume normal life if at all avoidable.

Practical Reasons to Babymoon
1. Allows both baby and family protection from illness. The baby's immune system has time to mature before being exposed to the general public.
2. Allows Mom to get familiar and comfortable with breast-feeding and baby care before she has to demonstrate in front of others.
3. Mother needs time for physical recovery and hormonal and emotional adjustment.
4. Mom will avoid overburdening abdominal and uterine muscles, thereby speeding recovery and decreasing the time it takes for her to return to a prepregnant state. Additionally, since lochia flow is heaviest during the first week, you eliminate dealing with that inconveniently.
5. Father and sibling(s) also benefit greatly from a babymoon. Everyone better understands the sacredness

and respect a new family member deserves. It also strengthens their bonds to the baby and mother. It's a gentle way of expanding the love in a family and helps to avoid jealousy. Love isn't always automatic, and a babymoon fosters that love and provides an opportunity for services toward the mother and baby. And it's well known that we end up loving those we serve.

With all this in mind, it's best to plan out your postpartum like you would your labor and birth. Not until about the past 100 years have women and families been without long-term postpartum help. When families began moving away from each other and birth moved into institutions, postpartum help became something available only to the wealthy. Hence postpartum depression and psychosis increased, the mother and baby couplet became more susceptible to illness and infection, and family bonds were stressed and weakened.

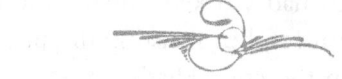

## What Should I Consider to Be Helped With and for How Long?

- Laundry
- Meals and cleanup afterward
- Light housekeeping (e.g., vacuuming, emptying trash, changing sheets, running errands)
- Care of siblings (taking them to school, etc.)
- Breast-feeding help
- Even if you have just the meals taken care of, that's a huge burden lifted. It's best to make up a schedule.
- A minimum of 1–2 weeks' help should be planned on. If you can get help for a full month, take it!

Caring for the baby should be your job. That's the whole point of postpartum help and babymooning. It's not so much a vacation as it is an opportunity to form strong, loving bonds. The couple should do all the bathing, feeding, diaper changing, etc. of the baby unless you are ill or recovering from a Cesarean.

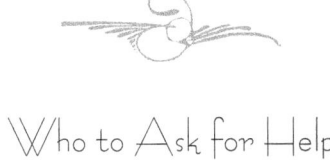

## Who to Ask for Help

- Family first, if available and supportive of your philosophy and parenting views. If there are teenage girls in your family, this is a great learning experience for them.
- Friends who are willing to do what they can when they can
- Support groups like church, Mommy and Me, La Leche League, etc.
- Professional help can include a postpartum doula

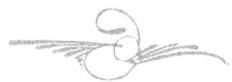

## Some Helpful Tips

- Request postpartum help as a gift instead of items you don't need for the baby; recommend that people pool money for a gift certificate for a postpartum doula.
- Ask for gift certificates for takeout or maid service.
- Make or purchase freezer meals ahead of time.
- Try to make the meals healthy; this also speeds recovery and allows for more energy.
- Get a cordless phone and caller ID (ask for it as a gift). Screen your calls.
- Set up a diaper changing station in multiple areas of the house.
- Relax and let things get messy. Your family will survive short term; it's more important to care for yourself and

the baby.
- Use paper plates and plastic silverware, etc instead of things that need washing.
- Breast-feeding can be much easier than bottle feeding in the long run once you cross those initial hurdles.
- Don't get out of your pajamas when people come by. It gives the impression that you don't need or want help. Do take a shower and sleep when you can, though.
- Don't be afraid to ask! If your friends and family really love you, they won't mind helping, and most of the time they truly want to help.

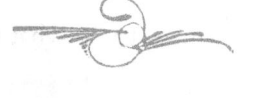

## Lessons From Jonelle's Postpartums

I have 5 children which were born over the span of 12 years. I was 21 when I had my first child, and 34 when I had my last. Let's just say that wisdom has come with time!

With my first child I had never heard of the idea of a baby moon. I worked up until a few days before my son was born, and despite a traumatic birth, was at church with him a few days after his birth. We even stopped at Toys R' Us on the way home from the hospital for a bouncy seat! Apparently, he really needed one to move forward in life. I do remember holding him a lot and cherishing those first six weeks. I resumed all my old tasks right away. This was not anything anyone imposed on me, but somehow I felt like this is what a "warrior woman" was, and I wanted to be that. Oh, how much I have learned!

With my second son, almost 3 years later, I had my first natural birth and that made a huge difference in my recovery, but still, I resumed life, going to church, cooking, cleaning and running errands, as I did before. I felt so good after this birth, I felt I "should" be doing these things. A week after he was born, though, I crashed. My body and mind said "no more", and I had to slow down. I got mastitis (a breastfeeding infection) soon after as a direct result. The difference this time was that I was not going back to work, but still felt I had to do it all.

My next birth, which was 4 ½ years later was so much different. By that time, I had been a doula and childbirth educator for some time. I had also begun my herbal studies and had done a lot of research on the postpartum time and how to truly make it heavenly. I had studied the birth traditions of Bali and other countries and found that the women were cherished and taken care of so well postpartum. Literally, there were barely any cases of postpartum depression. I was going to create my own Bali!

This birth experience was different though, namely because we were having twins. Also, it was to be our first homebirth. I took excellent care of myself this pregnancy because I wanted to go full term and have healthy babies at home. I had wonderful midwifery care, regular chiropractic adjustments and massages, ate and rested well. I had learned all about postpartum this time, and thought I was setting up an infallible infrastructure to make my postpartum magnificent!

I gave those who would be there certain tasks and roles. I sent a letter out to family and friends, asking for some privacy after birth, as we did not know how we would adjust with twins and all that came with our family growing from 2 to 4 children. A few meals had been set up, the house was clean, and I felt so prepared. The birth was short and beautiful, and at home. My healthy full term twins were amazing, and I could not be happier. I had not however factored in the postpartum after pains from a size 52 week uterus, getting the hang of tandem nursing, and being kind of in a haze. Even though I had intended to keep visitors to a minimum, many people still came, and I felt overwhelmed by it all.

I also was struggling to make sure our two older children were loved and taken care of. When the twins were 3 days old, our baby girl stopped eating and we had to go to the hospital for 3 long days of IV fluids as she crashed quickly and critically.

I was a zombie. I was in the hospital sitting on a lot of stitches from the birth, and trying to take care of one baby while aching for the health of another. It was at this point that I realized I had refused help when I should have accepted it. Left and right I had people willingly ask what we needed, and I told them all no. I could do this, we could do this and I was going to show the world my amazing mothering skills! What a huge mistake this was. I realize now how much help we needed, and stubbornness and pride kept me from accepting it. After returning home from the hospital, life resumed, the postpartum bubble was over, and life with 4 carried on. I felt gypped, to be honest. I had not even had a glance at a Bali experience!

Five and a half years later, I was pregnant with my 5th child. A singleton! I have heard from friends with twins how amazing it is to have just one baby after the twins, and how easy it is. I was looking forward to this. Also, my children were all at ages where they could easily attend to some of their most important needs. This time, I knew I needed the postpartum experience of my dreams. I also realized that no one was going to build it for me, that I had to set the wheels in motion to create it myself.

The first step was asking for help! Because I would be giving birth in my bedroom or bathroom, I wanted my room to feel like a haven. I asked two close friends to help me paint the room. This was no small task. It was to be a surprise for my husband who thought he had to do it. I also hung our pictures, my belly cast from our twins birth, and new bedspread. I sat in that room for the last few weeks leading up to this birth and literally absorbed the peace I felt in this room from the beauty I saw. I didn't just see freshly painted walls, I saw love and unconditional care for me from women who chose to serve me, and who I allowed to serve me!

My husband also had the opportunity to take a month off of work leading up to this birth. Now, I know that is a luxury, but it was enjoyed. He helped create this space with me, to enjoy and to take any pressures off of me to resume life as usual too soon. I belong to a freezer meal group, and had begun stock piling meals. By the time of Vaughn's birth, I had 24 freezer meals in my freezer. I remember I would open up that freezer just to behold the glory of them! It made me feel like my family was so taken care of and that their needs would be met. My dear sister came for a week before he was born. I had never had someone come to "help" me before a baby was born. She just came and said, "Tell me what to do. " I allowed her to cook, clean and make even more freezer meals. She also gave me a fantastic facial and massage. She entertained my kids and my husband and I as well. She even painted my toenails. It was wonderful!

    I had decided that I was not going to leave the comforts of my room with the baby until I felt ready. I had created a beautiful haven where everything I needed was there. My husband set up a small table in my room, and everything I could possibly need was there - A basket of lotion, gum, hair bands, my aromatherapy diffuser and all the herbal formulas and massage oils I would need for healing postpartum. I also had friends and family offer meals. I accepted! I was about two weeks overdue with this baby, and I was ready! His birth was wonderful and fast, and in the comforts of my favorite place- the tub. We chose just to have our children there with us and our beloved midwife. The house was alive with energy and anticipation.

    Right after the birth, the angels seemed to be present in every corner of every room. I felt heaven so peacefully and connected to those who had come before and those who were yet to come. I remember feeling literally on a celestial plane. My preparations and my surrendering to needing others had brought me to this state. There were no walls, no barriers to me being able to fully take this all in.

    After Vaughn was born, we enjoyed him with our family for a bit, and our midwife weighed him and snuggled him and me into bed together, we had the grandmas come. They came up to my room, (remember, I said I would not leave it), and they were able to enjoy and revel in his perfection. That night, with Vaughn tucked in between us, my husband and I fell into a blissful sleep. The next morning we awoke to 4 quiet and smiling faces, whispering what order they would like to hold him in. There we were a family of 7 all on our bed, and drinking in the ethereal and fleeting moments that a newborn brings.

 I slept, read, had food brought up to me, and occasionally got out of bed- but, only if I wanted to. The kids were free to come and go when I was awake. My husband would take the baby if I was asleep to snuggle with him, and bring him to me when he was hungry. For 7 straight nights we were lovingly brought meals, even lunch! Friends brought gifts, and thoughtful things such as homemade bath products for me and comfy pajamas. They even brought gifts for my other children. A dear, sweet friend brought a large tray of deli meats, cheeses, all the toppings and a huge basket of fresh rolls one afternoon. I felt so loved, my family's needs were being met, and we just felt cherished by it all. My mom brought my favorite bran muffins and soup the night he was born. She had had the muffin dough frozen in preparation. My mother in law came and quietly brought dinner, set the table, and fed my family. A dear sweet friend came and gave me a shoulder and back massage that was divine. Her husband made us a CD of songs from his extensive collection of various lullabies. I could really go on. It was beautiful.

 Now, I know this is not a common experience, but I can see how some preparations we made enhanced it. Like I said- allowing people to help and bring things and preparing the space. And, deciding to not leave the space!

 Every woman is different and so my experience may not be another's ideal, but it is a time that I think about often and it is a sacred memory to me. Slowly we emerged from our postpartum bubble, and resumed life, but it was at the pace we decided. That felt powerful and just right. This time will never happen again with this particular child. It is meant to be a time of wonder, a time of getting to know your baby, nursing on demand, and letting all the pregnancy hormones, settle and allowing peace to be more present. Here in the US we have an extremely high percentage of postpartum depression. Now that I look back, I feel I experienced a small degree of that with each of my previous children. I also know that my postpartum choices were largely a part of that. In Bali meals are brought for 40 days after. When you eat, other women or the father hold the baby, so you can eat easily. Women come and give massages daily. Your other children are attended to. Your only job is to nurse your baby. I know in this day, that many of these things may seem impossible. But let me propose that they aren't so farfetched. We just need to create them. I know that this time is vital to creating happy, calm mothers and in turn happy, peaceful babies, and families. My hope is for all women to experience a "Bali Postpartum Experience!"

# Afterword
## Can Peaceful Births Change the World?

The entirety of this chapter could be summed up in two words answering that question: Of course.

As I've outlined, it is clear that how well a pregnancy, birth, and postpartum go directly impacts how well parenting goes for both parents, and thus decides the upbringing of the child and, therefore, society. The roots of our being and character are developed at birth and through early childhood. It's not too farfetched to say that the roots are cultivated at conception and in utero. Even though we have the power to improve things along the way if we have experienced trauma at any stage of our existence, our lives and society would be far better off if those tools were given to us from the first moments of creation, rather than having to "dejunk" from the pain and injury that is inflicted on us.

We have an obligation to ourselves and our children to make the most gentle and peaceful decisions available. This, in turn, will create a peaceful parent, peaceful child, peaceful playground, peaceful adolescence, peaceful teen, peaceful young adult, peaceful adult, and a peaceful world. This isn't rocket science, and in fact its simplicity on the one hand makes it a collective reality. But on the other hand, people have been taught to complicate things and will often overlook the simple things in life because they've been programmed to believe by traumatized parents and elders that peace is hard to achieve and only afforded to the lucky few.

> *The influence of a vital woman vitalizes us.*
> —Joseph Campbell

Very few men will be seeking this out. I believe that it is our divine nature as women to do this. I pray that all men everywhere have this desire within them, but I feel it is our right as women to lead the way.

> *To help another human being reach one's potential is part of the divine mission of woman. As mother, teacher, or nurturing saint, she molds living clay to the shape of her hopes. In partnership with God, her divine mission is to help spirits live and souls be lifted. This is the measure of her creation. It is ennobling, edifying, and exalting.*[41]

For our sake and our children's sake, we cannot afford to base our decisions on fear or someone else's agenda but God's. You can do this, and do it joyfully. As a result, you will see the world around you begin to blossom into beauty and love. As you continue making decisions that support your higher good, you will experience this beauty and love on a consistent basis. This will inspire others around you to do the same.

This one act, of birthing peacefully, has within it the power to shape eternity. Do not trivialize or excuse away its importance. I've witnessed this one event mold mothers, fathers, and children into commanding, centered human beings or into fearful, angry human beings. I've also seen those once fearful and angry human beings transformed into the commanding and centered ones via a peaceful birth experience. How they all wish they could turn the clock back and spare themselves and their children suffering, though. And how it pains me to see people paralyzed by their birth trauma and stay in that pain for the rest of their lives. If they only knew the simplicity of steps to liberation from that pain. I think of my mother, my grandmothers, my sisters, my nieces and understand them more completely. Most of them hold onto the fear and the pain they have experienced in birth. I desperately want healing for them, but I have learned that that journey is one gained solely on their own. I can't do it for them, and I can't help them until and if they ever make the decision to heal. I can only pray that they are inspired by someone, somewhere to decide to knock on that door. I can only be there for them to help where they want help if they decide to walk through that door.

> *Loving people live in a loving world.*
> *Hostile people live in a hostile world.*
> *Same world.*
> —*Wayne Dyer*

All of us who live our lives on this frequency wish this for others. It's like finding a new religion. We want to tell others of "the good word." We do not wish to judge or be superior, but only to share in hopes of leading others to their peaceful paths. This way of being cannot be forced or coerced. It can only be achieved through modeling, mentoring, and example. It's quiet, yet speaks volumes far above any fearful yelling or clanking. But isn't that the pattern that truth and peace always follow? As we unravel our destructive DNA through love, compassion and gratitude, we can expect our own world, and the world around us to be at peace.

Here are the main points I want you to take away from this book:

1. Going in the direction of your desires can, and most often does, result in manifesting them, regardless of your present circumstances or barriers you see in your way. Are you going to just go along with what your mother, friend, mate, or caregiver wants for your birth and cross your fingers? Or are you going to prepare the soil, plant the seeds, and water and nurture your birth garden? It's all up to you. Choose what you want. Claim your birthright. You *can* do it.
2. Don't take no for an answer. If you don't have the caregiver you want, money you need, health you need, etc., don't settle. You can attain what you *want* and need, sometimes overnight. I have seen women change their RH- status to a positive one, couples have garage sales to raise money for their birth, and women change caregivers and intended birthplace, sometimes in the

midst of labor. There's very little you *can't* do.

3. Design your birth plans to serve you and your baby's highest interest, and no one else's. By eliminating outsiders'—even authority figures'—desires for your birth, you are not only increasing the odds of a peaceful, joyous birth, but are also increasing the odds of the safest birth possible.
4. Take inventory of all your abilities. Grab ahold of all your self-doubt and negative talk and say "buh-bye." You are smart, you are strong, you are or can be healthy, you are resourceful, you are intuitive, you are or can be properly cared for, and you are or can be supported.
5. The mind-spirit-body connection is real. You are a whole person, not a bag of muscle carrying a baby inside of it. What you think, hear, smell, every bit of it affects your physical self and progress, and therefore also affects your baby. Visualize your peaceful birth everyday from here on out. The way you birth does matter. The way you are treated does matter. What you are thinking does matter. Your perceptions and subsequent feelings do matter. Do not let this fact frighten you; rather, let it liberate you. You are not a victim of your body, your baby, your caregiver, your relationships, or your surroundings. You have the power to rise above that thinking.

I wish for you peace. Thank you for seeking it.

# Appendix
## A Brief History of Birth—How PABC Congealed

In order to gain an appreciation of how we got to our current state of affairs, how to improve the future of birth in this country for yourself and children, and also have a better understanding of this book, it's important that you get at least a brief overview of major events in birth history. Unless otherwise noted, all are U.S. events. See References for History of Birth Citations.

**Biblical times, African and European Continents:** Midwives adhered to a strict level of cleanliness per the admonition of Moses.[42] They also educated young women about their bodies, having children, and healthy pregnancies per that same admonition.

**AD 98** Soranus, a classical Roman who attended births, wrote a textbook of obstetrics that was used until the 16th century.

**Middle Ages and Renaissance (AD 500–1500), European Continent:** Barber-surgeons began trying to monopolize childbirth services. Women were forbidden to practice medicine or midwifery, and many midwives were accused of being witches and killed. Only men were allowed in the medical schools, and soon the barber-surgeon was delivering most of the babies.

**1522:** Dr. Wertt of Hamburg dressed up in women's clothes to gain entry to a labor room. He was discovered and burned at the stake for his efforts.

**1544:** The first book of obstetrics was printed in English called the *Birth of Mankynde* by Thomas Raynalde.

**1596:** Scipione Mercurio instructed attendants that for a Cesarean section, you need four strong assistants to hold the patient down as the incision is made; then apply a liquid concoction of varied herbs before removing the baby. He did not, however, record if this event would increase the odds that either the mother or child would survive.

**Colonial Times (circa AD 1600), European and North American Continent:** The importance of midwives to the social order is shown in the fact that several New England towns provided a house or lot rent-free to a midwife on condition that she does not refuse when called. Non-English colonies often kept midwives on the colonial payroll. In New Amsterdam they were called Zieckentroosters, or comforters of the sick, and received liberal salaries and special privileges. The Dutch West India Company salaried midwives and gave others free houses in the city on the explicit condition that they attend to the poor upon request. The French colony of Louisiana paid midwives until 1756 and provided physicians regularly to examine the quality of their practice.

**1600–1700:** Bishops in the Church of England were the first to legislate control over midwifery. Richard and Dorothy Wertz in the book *Lying-In* state:

> In the 17th century and before, English bishops were the only public authorities overseeing midwifery. The bishops had desired to prevent witchcraft associated with birth and to ensure that midwives were loyal to decrees of the church and state regarding birth, since midwives could baptize infants in emergencies. The bishops required that before beginning practice a midwife receive an Episcopal license, which prohibited her from coercing fees, giving abortifacients, practicing magic, or concealing information about birth events or parentages from civil or religious authorities. The license also prohibited her from refusing to attend poor women.[43]

Because of this influence, civil licensing began in the colonies. Again, quoting *Lying-In*:

> In the American colonies where the Anglican influence was most strongly felt, such as New York and Virginia,

civil licensing of midwives was required. In 1716 New York City required licensing for midwives in an ordinance that echoed the Episcopal licenses of England. Such licenses in effect placed the midwife in the role of servant of the state, a keeper of social and civil order.[44]

The predominant belief was that labor pain was woman's punishment for Eve's sins

**1650:** William Chaberlen invented forceps, but they were rarely used. They were instead kept as a family secret for many years.

**1697–1763:** William Smellie offered free care to indigent women, thus providing clinical teaching material.

**1700s:** Upper-class families began to rely on male doctors as primary caregivers

**1739–1791:** The first obstetric wards in Britain opened. Men became doctors merely by attending births and then being quizzed later.

**1750s–1880s:** Physicians did not associate hand washing with infection and would go from autopsies to delivering babies without washing in between.

**1765:** Dr. William Shippen opened the first formal training for midwives.

**1772:** 20 percent of delivered women contracted childbed fever, nearly all of whom died. Suggested causes: overcrowding, unwed maternity.

**1799:** Dr. Valentine Seaman led a course for midwives in New York City. A course in anatomy and midwifery was led by Dr. William Shippen in Philadelphia.

**1816:** The first stethoscope for listening to fetal heart tones externally was introduced by René T. H. Laënnec. Adapted stethoscopes, called Pinard horns and fetoscopes, became widely used.

**1817:** Britain mourns as Princess Charlotte dies five hours after a 50-hour labor and stillbirth. The public blamed her doctor, Dr. Croft, who later committed suicide. Opponents of man-midwifery advocated the return of female midwives. The medical establishment reacted by advocating quicker use of forceps.

**1828:** The word *obstetrician* was formed from the Latin, meaning "to stand before."

**1848:** Dr. Walter Channing of Boston first used ether for childbirth.

**1853:** Queen Victoria of England extolled the "virtues" of receiving chloroform during birth of her seventh baby. Receiving choloroform during childbirth became a status symbol.

**1860:** Louis Pasteur found bacteria and lack of washing was the major cause of puerperal (childbed) fever. Students were to scrub their hands in chloride of lime before having any contact with the patient. Physicians were the perpetuators of childbed fever, as midwives had observed the association between sanitation and maternal death thousands of years previous to this time.

**1894:** The first clinic Cesarean section was performed in Boston.

**1898:** German doctor August Bier injected cocaine into his assistant's spinal column (the forerunner of the modern day epidural). It numbed the fellow's lower body, but the next morning he woke with horrible vomiting and headaches.

**1900s:** Government involvement in maternity health care began in the early 1900s. Both federal and state bureaus became involved. The state bureaus primarily dealt with the problem of birth attendants. Even though fewer white, middle-class American women were being attended by midwives, many immigrants from Europe brought their own midwives with them and settled in major cities. As late as 1920 these midwives were attending 20–40 percent of all births in mid-Atlantic cities. In some cases, this meant they were practicing illegally. Fewer than 5 percent of women gave birth in hospitals.

**1902–1960s:** Scopolamine, which causes amnesia, was used during childbirth.

**1910:** The Flexner Report revealed that 90 percent of doctors were without a college education. The Carnegie Foundation for the Advancement of Teaching published Abraham Flexner's critical report on medical education in North America. Flexner stated that obstetrics made "the very worst showing."

**1914:** New England Twilight Sleep Association was founded to force hospitals to offer the procedure. Upper-class women formed Twilight Sleep Societies, and it became a sign of superiority to use it during childbirth. Twilight Sleep is a combination of morphine, for relief of pain, and scopolamine, an amnesiac that caused women to have no memories of giving birth. Upper-class women initially welcomed it as a symbol of medical progress, although its negative effects were later publicized.

**1914–late 1960s:** Ankle and wrist restraints were used to keep women from injuring themselves under the influence of Twilight Sleep.

**1915:** A paper by Joseph DeLee in the Association for the Study and Prevention of Infant Mortality described childbirth as a pathological process. He stated that childbirth was not a normal function and that midwives had no place in childbirth.

**1915–1929:** Infant mortality from birth injuries increased by 40–50 percent. Between 30-50% of women gave birth in hospitals by 1921.

**1918:** The United States stood 17th out of 20 nations in mortality rates. Maternal mortality reached a plateau, with a high of 6 to 7 deaths per 1,000 births between 1900 and 1930.

**1920:** The medical profession won stronger licensing laws and helped shape the medical system so that its structure supported, rather than undermined, professional dominion. Forceps were used in 30 percent of births. The most frequently used obstetric textbook, by Dr. Joseph DeLee, stated that childbirth is a pathological process from which few escape "damage." In efforts to prevent problems, he proposed that the caregiver employ routine interventions. He suggested that the obstetrician sedate women at the beginning of labor, allow the cervix to dilate, give ether during the pushing stage, cut an episiotomy, deliver the baby with forceps, extract the placenta, give medications for the uterus to contract, and repair the episiotomy. Because of his influence with the American obstetrician, caring for labor and birthing women went from responding to problems as they arose to attempting to prevent problems through routine use of interventions as a way to control the course of labor. This led to every woman in labor being dealt with in this way. To a large extent, American obstetrics is still functioning under the medical paradigm of childbirth it inherited from Dr. DeLee.

**1920s:** Moving birth into the hospital removed a trained female attendant and the benefits.

**1921:** The Sheppard-Tower and Infancy Protection Act became law. It provided funds to train people to seek for ways to improve maternal and child health. A range of 30–50 percent of women gave birth in hospitals.

**1925:** Mary Breckenridge founded the Frontier Nursing Service of Hyden, Kentucky.

**1929:** The American Medical Association lobbied against the Sheppard-Tower Act and Congress allowed it to expire.

**1930:** The American Board of Obstetricians and Gynecology was established. Obstetricians sought to achieve dominance over the nonphysician specialists, such as midwives. Nurse-midwifery appears, stemming from the profession of nursing rather than midwifery. Their emphasis was on assisting doctors in their profession. Nurse-midwives provided supervision for rural immigrant midwives. Most practicing midwives were black or poor-white granny midwives working in the rural South. A scholar who conducted an intensive study concluded that the 41 percent increase in infant mortality due to birth injuries between 1915 and 1929 was due to obstetrical interference in birth.

**1933:** Maternal mortality was 58.1 deaths per 1,000. Maternal mortality had not declined between 1915 and 1930 in spite of women moving childbirth into hospitals, increased prenatal care, and better birthing techniques as reported by the White House Conference on Child Health.

**1935:** 37 percent of births occur in hospitals.

**1938:** Twilight Sleep used in all hospital births.

**1939:** 50 percent of all women (75 percent of all urban women) delivered in hospitals.

**1940:** 95 percent Twilight Sleep rate. This heavy dose of narcotics and amnesiacs completely incapacitated laboring women and caused women to lose control. Maternal mortality is 47 deaths per 1,000.

**1944:** Dr. Grantley Dick-Reed wrote *Childbirth without Fear.*

**1950:** 88 percent of births occurred in hospitals. Maternal mortality was 29.2 deaths per 1,000. Forceps were used 75 percent of the time.

**1953:** Dr. Fernand Lamaze published his findings about labor and delivery in Russia. His work helped bring the fathers back into the birth room.

**1955:** The American College of Nurse Midwives (ACNM) was formed.

**1956:** La Leche League was founded.

**1958:** Dr. Robert Bradley introduced husband-coached natural childbirth

**1957:** The book *Thank You, Dr. Lamaze* by Marjorie Karmel was published

**1960:** Marjorie Karmel and one of her book's admirers, Elisabeth Bing, a clinical assistant professor at New York Medical College, formed the American Society for Psychoprophylaxis in Obstetrics (better known as ASPO/Lamaze), to teach childbirthing classes. 97 percent of births occurred in hospitals. Maternal mortality was 26 deaths per 1,000. Continuous electronic fetal monitoring was introduced.

**1963:** International Childbirth Education Association (ICEA) was founded.

**1965:** On July 30 U.S. President Lyndon B. Johnson signed into effect Medicaid and Medicare.

**1968:** Continuous electronic fetal monitoring was introduced, only used on 5–10 percent of women, those considered "high risk."

**1970s and onward:** Doctors made more money per hour for a hospital visit than they did for an office visit.

**1970:** Maternal mortality is 20 deaths per 1,000. National certification in nurse-midwifery educational programs began.

**1970–1971:** HMOs were created.

**1971:** The Farm, a hippie commune in Tennessee, was founded by Stephen and Ina May Gaskin, the mother of modern midwifery. The Birth Center of Santa Cruz was started.

**1973:** ACNM stated, "The preferred site for childbirth because of the distinct advantage to the physical welfare is the hospital."

**1975:** The Birth Collective at Freemont Women's Clinic in Seattle began. Less than 1 percent of births were attended by midwives. Maternal mortality was 16.1 deaths per 1,000. 20 percent of American women chose to have an epidural.

**1976:** The Division of Nursing began to fund nurse-midwifery education programs. 5 percent Cesarean rate.

**1977:** Informed Homebirth (IH) was founded by Rahima Baldwin Dancy in response to the need for information on how to prepare for a safe delivery at home. The original childbirth educator training program was developed in 1978.

**1979:** The first studies were conducted on labor anesthesia, including Demerol.

**1980:** 98.9 percent of births occurred in hospitals. The ACNM developed guidelines for establishing "alternative" birthing services. They changed their negative home birth statement to one that endorsed practice in all settings. Maternal mortality was 12.6 deaths per 1,000. The American Academy of Family Physicians (AAFP) opposed nurse-midwifery and issued formal statements to that effect. AAFP stated the belief that all nurse-midwives should work nonindependently and that all payments should go through the physician.

**1982:** The Midwives Alliance of North America (MANA) began. One-third of its members were CNMs, and the rest were other types of midwives. Insurance (liability) coverage declined rapidly for CNMs from 1982 to 1985, with some companies either totally withdrawing from coverage or making it expensive. 16 percent of all births occur on Saturdays and 16.6 percent of births occur on Sundays.

**1983:** The National Association of Childbearing Centers was established. The Federal Trade Commission intervened in a CNM-doctor case and negotiated an agreement that prohibited the insurance company from any form of discrimination against doctors who collaborate with CNMs.

**1985:** The AMA set out to create legislation and regulation for all nonphysician health-care workers that would not allow these workers to practice independently. Maternal mortality was 10.6 deaths per 1,000. 6.8 percent of babies are born with low birth weight (under 2,500 g). The World Health Organization (WHO) recommends that the Cesarean section rate should not be higher than 10–15 percent.

**1988:** 25 percent Cesarean rate. Patient-controlled epidurals, which allow women in labor to adjust the timing and frequency of their anesthesia with the push of a button, come on the scene.

**1989:** Forceps used in 5.5 percent of births. 18.9 VBAC rate; 9 percent induction rate. 47.7 percent of women received at least one ultrasound during pregnancy. 8 percent Continuous Electronic Fetal Monitoring rate. 9.4 percent of births occurred prior to 37 weeks gestation.

**Late 1980s:** Hospitals introduced LDR rooms (Labor, Delivery and Recovery rooms, where you labored, gave birth in, and recovered all in the same room rather than moving to different rooms for each of those stages).

**1990:** 10.7 percent of births occurred prior to 37 weeks gestation. Physicians who at one time had no interest in taking care of poor, pregnant women became more willing to do so as Medicaid increased payouts for services and made acquiring these fees easier. 41 percent of births occurred between 37–40 weeks gestation. Once again, AAFP opposed nurse-midwifery and issued formal statements to that effect. AAFP stated the belief that all nurse-midwives should work nonindependently and that all payments should go through the physician. Maternal mortality is 9.2 deaths per 1,000. 11.3 percent of births occur at or beyond 42 weeks' gestation. 75.8 percent of women received prenatal care.

**1992:** Forceps used 10 percent of the time. Doulas of North America (DONA) was founded to legitimize the benefits of female birth attendants. The governor of New York signed a new Professional Midwifery Practice Act into law in July. The act defined midwifery as a profession with a specific scope of practice and called for a board of midwifery to regulate the profession.

**1992–1999:** A handful of organizations are founded to train and certify independent childbirth educators and doulas.

**1993:** Again, the AAFP opposed nurse-midwifery and issued formal statements to that effect. AAFP stated the belief that all nurse-midwives should work nonindependently and that all payments should go through the physician. The first randomized, controlled trial to observe the effects of epidural anesthesia was halted after it was concluded that it would be unethical to continue the study due to bad outcomes. The ACNM obtained a stable, long-term professional liability program. The number of jurisdictions that grant prescriptive authority to CNMs increased from 14 in 1984 to 31 in 1995.

**1994:** 94.5 percent of births occurred in hospitals. There was a 14.7 percent induction rate and 85 percent continuous EFM rate. The North American Registry of Midwives (NARM) offered its first written examination to test the knowledge needed for safe, beginning-level, direct-entry midwifery practice to implement a process to certify direct-entry midwives. Federal law required all state Medicaid programs to pay for care provided by CNMs.

**1995:** 21 percent Cesarean rate. Maternal mortality is 7.6 deaths per 1,000. Some insurance companies refused to write policies for physicians who worked with midwives—or charged physicians higher premiums if they did—thus imposing restrictions and requirements that limited and burdened the practice.

**1996:** NARM expands the certification process to include entry-level midwives. 28.3 percent VBAC rate

**1998:** 19.4 percent induction rate

**1998:** The rate of midwife-attended births grew at a high and rising rate, showing a 45 percent increase since 1982. The rate of midwife-attended hospital births rose even more sharply, increasing by 1,000 percent since 1975.

**1999:** 6 percent forceps rate. VBAC rates plummet after ACOG releases new guidelines for doctors and hospitals attending VBACs, making it unrealistic for either of them to support VABCs, both financially and in practice. Dr. Marsden Wagner (former director of Women's and Children's Health in the WHO) noted that ACOG "has no data to support it [the 1999 VBAC recommendations], no studies showing improvements in maternal mortality or perinatal mortality related to the characteristics of institutions or availability of physicians."

**2000:** Maternal mortality is 6.9 deaths per 1,000. Much to the chagrin of ACOG and most OBs and hospitals, findings on a landmark study on using CPMs for home birth is released showing that home births with a qualified midwife are safer than OB- or CNM-assisted hospital births.

**2001:** 11.9 percent of births occurred before 37 weeks gestation. 16.4 VBAC rate

**2002:** 26.1 percent cesarean rate. 20.6 percent induction rate. 85 percent Continuous EFM rate. 91.3 percent of births occurred in hospitals. Maternal mortality is 7.1 deaths per 1,000. 7.8 percent of infants are born with low birth weight (under 2,500 g). 12.1 percent of births occurred before 37 weeks gestation. 51 percent of births occurred between 37–41 weeks gestation. 6.7 percent occur at or beyond 42 weeks gestation. 12.6 percent VBAC rate. Midwives attend 8.1 percent of all births (94.6 percent CNM attended). 83.7 percent of women received prenatal care. Of all out-of-hospital births, 65 percent occurred at home and 27 percent occurred at a free-standing birth center. 68 percent of pregnant women received at least one ultrasound during pregnancy. Births occurring by day of the week:

| Saturday: | 8,573 |
| Sunday: | 7,526 |
| Monday: | 11,453 |
| Tuesday: | 12,823 |
| Wednesday: | 12,083 |
| Thursday: | 12,365 |
| Friday: | 12,283 |

**2003:** 26.1 percent Cesarean rate. 11 percent of vaginal births are attended by certified nurse-midwives. Direct-entry, CPM, and lay midwives attend 4 of every 1,000 U.S. births. The U.S. ranks 41 out of 60 nations in infant mortality.

**2004:** Maternal mortality is 7 deaths per 1,000

**2005:** WHO and UNICEF rank the U.S. 34th in maternal mortality. AAFP reviewed all of the evidence on VBAC and the necessity of 24-hour OB and anesthesia, it recommended that "TOLAC (trial of labor after Cesarean) should not be restricted only to facilities with available surgical teams present throughout labor since there is no evidence that these additional resources result in improved outcomes."

**2006:** 22 percent of women have their labors induced.

**2007:** 31.8 percent Cesarean rate, representing a more than 50 percent increase since 1996.

**2008:** 33 percent Cesarean rate. The United States has some of the worst pregnancy outcomes than almost every other industrialized country, yet provides the world's most expensive maternity care. An average 80 percent of women elect for an epidural for vaginal delivery. ACOG releases the following statement after much press is given to the Ricki Lake documentary *The Business of Being Born*:

> The American College of Obstetricians and Gynecologists (ACOG) reiterates its long-standing opposition to home births. . . . ACOG acknowledges a woman's right to make informed decisions regarding her delivery and to have a choice in choosing her health care provider, but ACOG does not support programs that advocate for, or individuals who provide, home births. Childbirth decisions should not be dictated or influenced by what's fashionable, trendy, or the latest cause célèbre.

**2009:** America ranks 45th in Infant Mortality rankings. ACOG revises its guidelines on electronic fetal monitoring, denouncing years of standard practice. According to Dr. George A. Macones, who headed the development of the ACOG document:

> Since 1980, the use of EFM has grown dramatically, from being used on 45% of pregnant women in labor to 85% in 2002, Although EFM is the most common obstetric procedure today, unfortunately it hasn't reduced perinatal mortality or the risk of cerebral palsy. In fact, the rate of cerebral palsy has essentially remained the same since World War II despite fetal monitoring and all of our advancements in treatments and interventions."

In another ACOG revision, they stated that elective inductions should not be done prior to 39 weeks gestation and that the physician capable of performing a Cesarean should be readily available any time induction is used in the event that the induction isn't successful in producing a vaginal delivery, although they do not define what "readily available" means.

ACOG admits decades of inappropriate guidelines when they relax their position on women eating and drinking in labor. Once completely banned during labor and birth, they now support women drinking "modest amounts of clear liquids during labor if they wish," citing that they now see the benefits of eating and drinking during labor in relation to providing energy and comfort.

As you can see, childbirth has not always been viewed as a peaceful experience and has always been subject to predominant cultural attitudes, whether those voices are from the religious, scientific, or public and social sector. It can be easy to get wrapped up in the pain, fear, and other obvious factors that can accompany childbirth. But it takes a deep understanding of ourselves, faith in the process and our bodies and babies, and a long-term perspective to walk into the birth experience with confidence and eagerness and walk out of it with the joy and serenity you are seeking. We are at a distinct advantage in our earth's history where we have thousands of years of both successful and failed documented birth practices, the knowledge of how to prevent the majority of complications in pregnancy, birth and postpartum, the experience and wisdom of our ancestors and modern-day birth "sages." There is all kinds of support during the birth year, and science and technology to back us up where we need it, such that there is no need to fear the birth process as our mothers before us did. We should be rejoicing and throwing off the old robes of the fear of pain or being conscious for the event, the distrust of our bodies, babies, and instincts, the patriarchal (from religion or government) control of this process, and the mind-set that it is better, clinically or otherwise, to completely hand our bodies and babies over to "the experts" to handle. For too long we have handed over our responsibility and power to those who would willingly shape our lives for us. Birth transforms you into much more than a mother. Birth is a rite of passage. It is *your* right of passage. Claim it!

> All occurrences of violence, negativity, et cetera in any society are the expression of stress in the collective consciousness.
> —Maharishi Mahesh Yogi

## Footnotes

1 Sykes, 2001
2 Elias, 2002
3 McRae et al., 2004
4 Bohm, 1989; Chester, 1987
5 Lipton, 2005
6 Crawford, 2007
7 Menacker, 2010
8 Campero L., 1995; Keenan P., 2000; Kennell J, 1991; Klaus MH, 1997; Langer A, 1998; Nolan M., 1995; Scott KD., 1999; Zhang J., 1996
9 http://www.rainbowbody.net/Ongwhehonwhe/cherokee.htm
10 Johnson, AP/USA Today, 5/4
11 Orme-Johnson, D. W.,, 1988
12 Grady, 2010
13 Northrup, 1998, pp. 493, 494.
14 Lipton, 2005
15 Lipton, 2005
16 McCraty, R., 2003
17 Crawford, 2007
18 See References
19 UNICEF, 2005
20 Goer, 1995; emphasis added
21 Goer, 1995
22 Soucy, Dionne, & Dionne, 1997
23 Saturday Night Live, 2006-2007
24 Scheibner, 1993

[25] Courois & Courtois, 1992, pp. 22–223; Fraser & Boulvain, 1996, pp. 1125–1131; Hanson, 2003, p. 93; Harger, 2003, p. 205; Tallman & Hering, 1998, 19–21; USDHHS, 2003

[26] Kitzinger, 2001, pp. 188, 189; Englemann, 2009, p. 23; Sutton, 1995, p. 11; Balaskas, 1992, p. 139; Davis-Floyd, 1992, p. 122; Odent, 1994, p. 47

[27] Prentice and Lind, 1987 p 1375-1377

[28] *Obstetric Myths vs. Research Realities*, Goer 1995

[29] Perez, P., 2000, Goer, H., 1995, Wagner, MG., 1994, Obstetrics and Gynecology, May 2005, BMJ, November 1990

[30] Burn & Greenish, 1992, pp. 47–49; Garland & Jones, 1997, p. 371; Erikkson et al., 1996, pp. 642–644; Favero, 1986, p. 283

[31] Perez, P., 2000, Goer, H., 1995, Wagner, MG., 1994, Obstetrics and Gynecology, May 2005, BMJ, November 1990

[32] CTV, 2004; Paediatric and Perinatal Epidemiology 2007; *The Associated Press*, January 12, 2010

[33] National Vital Statistics Report, 2007

[34] Johnson & Daviss, 2005

[35] Cahill et al., 2010

[36] *The Journal of Neuroscience, 2006.*

[37] Chiras, 2003

[38] *European Journal of Social Psychology, 2009*

[39] Begley, 2008

[40] Godin, 2008, p. 64

[41] Nelson, 1989, p. 22

[42] Atkinson, 1956, p 20; The Bible, Leviticus 12-15, Numbers 19:11-22

[43] Wertz & Wertz, 1989, pp 6-7

[44] Wertz & Wertz, 1989. p 7

# References

The Associated Press (*2010, January 12*) "C-section rates around globe at 'epidemic' levels" Retrieved from http://news.ca.msn.com/top-stories/msnbc-article.aspx?cp-documentid=23241689

Atkinson, DT. (1956). *Magic, Myth and Medicine.* Cleveland, OH: World Pub. Co.

BBC (2000), "Born Above the Floodwaters". Retrieved from http://www.literacytools.ie/files/pdfs/MiracleBaby.pdf

Balaskas, J. (1992). *Active birth.* Boston, MA: Harvard Common Press.

Begley, S. (2008) *Train your mind, change your brain.* New York: Ballantine Books.

Betrán, AP., Merialdi, M., Lauer, JA., Bing-Shun, W., Thomas, J., Van Look, P., Wagner, W., (2007) "Rates of caesarean section: analysis of global, regional and national estimates" *Paediatric and Perinatal Epidemiology 21* (2): 98 – 113.

The Bible, Leviticus 12-15, Numbers 19:11-22

Bohm, D. (1989). *Quantum theory.* Mineola, N.Y.: Dover Publications.

Burn, E., & Greenish, K. (1992). "Pooling information." *Nursing Times 89*(8): 47–49.

Cahill, A., Tuuli, M., Odibo, A., Stamilio, D., & Macones, G. (2010). "Vaginal birth after Caesarean for women with three or more prior Caesareans: Assessing safety and success." *BJOG.* doi: 10.1111/j.1471-0528.2010.02498.x

Chester, M. (1987). *Primer of quantum mechanics.* Mineola, N.Y.: Dover Publications.

Chiras, D. D. (2003) *Human body systems: Structure, function and environment.* Sudbury, MA: Jones and Bartlett Publishers

Courtois, C., & Courtois, R. C. (1992). "Pregnancy and childbirth as triggers for abuse memories: Implications for Care." *Birth 19*(4), 22–223.

Crawford, A. (2007). *The Nature of God.* Bloomington, Indiana: Trafford Publishing.

CTV (2004, April 21). "Canada's Caesarean section rate highest ever". Retrieved from http://www.ctv.ca/servlet/ArticleNews/story/CTVNews/20040421/caesarean_rate_040421?s_name=&no_ads=.

Davis-Floyd, R. (1992) *Birth as an American rite of passage.* Los Angeles, CA: University of California Press Berkeley.

Englemann, G. J. (2009), *Labor among primitive peoples.* Charleston, SC: BiblioLife.

Elias, M. (2002, July 7). "Study: Antidepressant barely better than placebo." *USA Today.* Retrieved from http://www.usatoday.com/news/health/drugs/2002-07-08-antidepressants.htm

Erikkson, M., et al. (1996, August.). "Warm tub bath during labor: A study of 1,385 women with prelabor rupture of the membranes after 34 weeks of gestation." *Acta Obstetricia et Gynecologieca Scandinavica 75*(7): 642–644.

Favero, M. (1986). "Risk of AIDS and other STDs from swimming pools and whirlpools is nil." *Postgraduate Medicine 80*(1):283.

Althaus, Dr. Jayne "Fetal heart fails to signal cerebral palsy risk." (2004, March) Society for Gynecologic Investigation Annual Meeting, Houston, Texas

Fraser, W., & Boulvain, M. (1996). "Induction of labour: indications and methods." *Journal SOGC.* 18:1125–1131.

Garland, D., & Jones, K. (1997, June). "Waterbirth: Updating the evidence." *British Journal of Midwifery 5*(6): 371.

Godin, S. (2008). *Tribes.* New York: Penguin Books.

Goer, H. (1995). *Obstetric Myths vs. Research Realities.* Westpoint, CT: Bergin & Garvey.

Grady, D., (March 6, 2010). "Lessons At An Indian Hospital About Birth." *New York Times.* Retrieved from http://www.nytimes.com/2010/03/07/health/07birth.html

Hanson, S. (2003, Summer). "To VE or not to VE? That is the question." Association of Radical Midwives: 97.

Harger, J. H. (2003, January). "Cerclage and cervical insufficiency: an evidence-based analysis." *Obstetrics & Gynecology, 101*(1), 205.

Jacobson, B., Nyberg, K., Grönbladh, L., Eklund, G., Bygdeman, M., Rydberg, U., (1990). "Opiate addiction in adult offspring through possible imprinting after obstetric treatment," *BMJ* 301:1067-1070

Johnson, AP/USA Today, 5/4 Retrieved from http://www.msnbc.msn.com/id/7722862/

Johnson, K. C., & Daviss, B-A. (2005) "Outcomes of planned home births with certified professional midwives: large prospective study in North America." *BMJ* 330:1416

Kitzinger S. (2001). *Rediscovering birth.* New York, NY: Atria.

Klaus, M. H., Kennell, J. H., & Klaus, P. H. (1993). *Mothering the mother.* New York, NY: Perseus Books.

Korte, D., & Scaer, R. M. (1992). *A good birth, a safe birth* (3rd ed.). Boston, MA: Harvard Common Press.

Lally, P., Van Jaarsveld, C.H.M., Potts, H.W.W., Wardle, J., "How Are Habits Formed: Modeling habit formation in the real world", *European Journal of Social Psychology, 2009*

Lieberman, E., Davidson, K., Lee-Parritz, A., Shearer, E., "Changes in Fetal Position During Labor and Their Association With Epidural Analgesia", *Obstetrics and Gynecology, May 2005*

Lipton, B. (2005). *The Biology of Belief.* New York: Hay House.

Menacker, F., Hamilton, BE., "Recent Trends in Cesarean Delivery in the United States", NCHS data brief, no 35. Hyattsville, MD: National Center for Health Statistics. 2010.

McCraty, R., M., D., "Modulation of DNA Conformation by Heart-Focused Intention," Research Center, Publication No. 03-008. *Institute of HeartMath, 2003*

McRae, C., Cherin, E., Yamazaki, T. G., Diem, G., Vo, A. H., Russell, D., et al. (2004). "Effects of perceived treatment on quality of life and medical outcomes in a double-blind placebo surgery trial." *Archives of General Psychiatry, 61,* 412–420.

Nelson, R. M. (1989, November). "Woman—of infinite worth," *Ensign.*

Northrup, C. (1998). *Women's bodies, women's wisdom.* New York: Bantam Books.

*Journal of Perinatal Education* (16)1, 32S–64S.

Odent, M. (1994). *Birth reborn.* Medford, NJ: Birth Works Press

Orme-Johnson, D. W., Alexander, C. N., Davies, J. L., Chandler, H. M., & Larimore, W. E. (1988). "International peace project in the Middle East: The effects of the Maharishi Technology of the Unified Field."

*Journal of Conflict Resolution, 32*(4), 776–812.)

Perez., P., Snedeker, C., (2000). *Special Women.* Johnson, VT: Cutting Edge Press.

Prentice, A., Lind, T., "Fetal heart rate monitoring during labor-too frequent intervention, too little benefit?" *Lancet 1987;2*: 1375-1377

Saturday Night Live (2006-2007), "Penelope the Party Pooper," *NBC*, Season 32, Episode 16

Schaefer A, Braver TS, Reynolds JR, Burgess GC, Yarkoni T, Gray JR (2006), "Individual differences in amygdala activity predict response speed during working memory." *The Journal of Neuroscience* 26:10120–8

Scheibner, V., (1993) *Vaccination 100 Years of Orthodox Research shows that Vaccines Represent a Medical Assault on the Immune System.* UK: Minerva Books

Soucy, J. Y., Dionne, Y., & Dionne, C. (1997) *Family secrets: The Dionne quintuplets' autobiography.* New York, NY: Berkley Books.

Sutton, J., & Scott, P. (1995). Understanding and Teaching Optimal Foetal Positioning. Tauranga, New Zealand: Birth Concepts.

Sykes, B. (2001). *The Seven Daughters of Eve.* New York: W. W. Norton & Company.

Tallman, N., & Hering, C. (1998). "Child abuse and its effects on birth." *Midwifery Today,* 45:19–21.

UNICEF. (2005). WHO/UNICEF/UNFPA/The World Bank Estimates of Maternal Mortality 2005. Retrieved from http://www.childinfo.org/maternal_mortality_countrydata.php

Wagner, MG. (1994). *Pursuing the Birth Machine.* Naperville, IL: ACE Graphics

Wertz, R. W., & Wertz, D. C. (1989). *Lying-in.* New Haven, CT: Yale University Press.

Williamson, M. (1992). *A return to love.* New York: HarperCollins.

**Doula Studies**

Campero L, García C, Díaz C, Ortiz O, Reynoso S, Langer A. "Alone, I wouldn't have known what to do: a qualitative study on social support during labor and delivery in Mexico." *Soc Sci Med 1998 Aug 47*:3 395-403.

Barron SP, Lane HW, Hannan TE, Struempler B, Williams JC. "Factors influencing duration of breast feeding among low-income women." *J Am Diet Assoc 1988 Dec 88*:12 1557-61.

Keenan P., "Benefits of massage therapy and use of a doula during labor and childbirth." *AlternTher Health Med 2000 Jan;6*:66-74.

Kennell J, Klaus M, McGrath S, Robertson S, Hinkley C., "Continuous emotional support during labor in a US hospital. A randomized controlled trial." *JAMA 1991 May 1 265*:17 2197-201

Klaus MH, Kennell JH., "The doula: an essential ingredient of childbirth rediscovered." *Acta Paediatr 1997 Oct 86*:10 1034-6.

Langer A, Campero L, Garcia C, Reynoso S., "Effects of psychosocial support during labour and childbirth on breastfeeding, medical interventions, and mothers' well-being in a Mexican public hospital: a randomised clinical trial." *Br J Obstet Gynaecol 1998 Oct 105*:10 1056-63.

Manning-Orenstein G., "A birth intervention: the therapeutic effects of Doula support versus Lamaze preparation on first-time mothers' working models of caregiving." *Altern Ther Health Med 1998 Jul 4*:4 73-81.

Nolan M., "Supporting women in labour: the doula's role." *Mod Midwife 1995 Mar 5*:3 12-5.

Gordon NP, Walton D, McAdam E, Derman J, Gallitero G, Garrett L., "Effects of providing hospital-based doulas in health maintenance organization hospitals." *Obstet Gynecol 1999 Mar 93*:3 422-6.

Scott KD, Berkowitz G, Klaus M., "A comparison of intermittent and continuous support during labor: a meta-analysis." *Am J Obstet Gynecol 1999 May 180*:5 1054-9.

Scott KD, Klaus PH, Klaus MH., "The obstetrical and postpartum benefits of continuous support during childbirth." *J Womens Health Gend Based Med 1999 Dec;8*:1257-64.

Wang D, Mao X, Qian S. (1997) "Clinical observation on Doula delivery." *Zhonghua Fu Chan Ke Za Zhi* 32:11 659-61. Retrieved from http://www.ncbi.nlm.nih.gov/pubmed/9639765.

Zhang J, Bernasko JW, Leybovich E, Fahs M, Hatch MC., "Continuous labor support from labor attendant for primiparous women: a meta-analysis." *Obstet Gynecol 1996 Oct 88*:4 Pt 2 739-44

Raphael D., "Support and variation, the needs of the breast-feeding woman." *Acta Paediatr Jpn 1989 Aug 31*:4 369-72.

**History of Birth Citations**

The Editors of Time-Life Books. (1998, Nov.). *Events that Shaped the Century*. Time Life.

Rooks, J P. (1999). *Midwifery and Childbirth in America*. Philadelphia, PA: Temple University Press

Starr, Paul. (1984). *The Social Transformation of American Medicine.* New York, NY: Basic Books.

U.S. News and World Report. (1973). *200 Years: A Bicentennial Illustrated History of the United States.*

Wertz, RW., Wertz, DC., *Lying-In: A History of Childbirth in America.* 1989 New Haven, CT: Yale University Press.

Evans, J., "Induction rate doubled in the U.S. from 1990 to 1998". *J. Reprod. Med. 47[2]*:120-24, 2002. Retrieved from http://findarticles.com/p/articles/mi_m0CYD/is_9_37/ai_85591457/?tag=content;col1

National Vital Statistics Report, Volume 52, Number 10. *Births: Final Data for 2002.* Retrieved from http://www.cdc.gov/nchs/data/nvsr/nvsr52/nvsr52_10.pdf

National Vital Statistics Report, Volume 57, Number 12. *Births: Preliminary Data for 2007.* Retrieved from http://www.cdc.gov/nchs/data/nvsr/nvsr57/nvsr57_12.pdf

Rooks, J P (1997), *Midwifery & Childbirth in America.* Philadelphia, PA: Temple University Press

Cassidy, T., *Taking Great Pains.* Retrieved from http://wondertime.go.com/learning/article/childbirth-pain-relief.html

CIA World Factbook, *Country Comparison: Infant mortality rate.* Retrieved from https://www.cia.gov/library/publications/the-world-factbook/rankorder/2091rank.html

United States, Central Intelligence Agency. *The 2003 CIA World Factbook*

UNICEF (United Nations Children's Fund). 2005. WHO/UNICEF/UNFPA/The World Bank Estimates of Maternal Mortality 2005. Retrieved from http://www.childinfo.org/maternal_mortality_countrydata.php

World Health Organization. "Appropriate technology for birth". *Lancet* 1985; 2: 436-7.

Johnson, KC, *Outcomes of planned home births with certified professional midwives: large prospective study in North America"* BMJ 2005;330:1416 (18 June). Retrieved from http://www.bmj.com/cgi/content/full/330/7505/1416

ACOG Statement on Home Births, February 6, 2008. Retrieved from http://www.acog.org/from_home/publications/press_releases/nr02-06-08-2.cfm

Wall, E., Roberts, R., Deutchman, M., Hueston, W., Atwood, LA., Ire-

land, B., *"Trial of Labor After Cesarean (TOLAC), Formerly Trial of Labor Versus Elective Repeat Cesarean Section for the Woman With a Previous Cesarean Section."*
AAFP Policy Action March 2005. Retrieved from http://www.aafp.org/online/etc/medialib/aafp_org/documents/clinical/clin_recs/tolacpolicy.Par.0001.File.dat/clinicalrec_tolac.pdf

Wagner, M., "What Every Midwife Should Know About ACOG and VBAC: Critique of ACOG Practice Bulletin No. 5, July 1999, "Vaginal Birth After Previous Cesarean Section". Retrieved from http://www.midwiferytoday.com/articles/acog.asp

ACOG, *"ACOG Issues Revision of Labor Induction Guidelines"*. & Gynecology, Practice Bulletin #107, "Induction of Labor," August 2009. Retrieved from http://www.acog.org/from_home/publications/press_releases/nr07-21-09.cfm

ACOG, *"Recommendations Relax on Liquid Intake during Labor"*. & Gynecology, Committee Opinion #441, "Oral Intake during Labor," September 2009. Retrieved from http://www.acog.org/from_home/publications/press_releases/nr08-21-09-2.cfm

Banks, A C (1999). *Birth Chairs, Midwives and Medicine*, Lanham, MD: University Press

Cutter, IS., Viets, HR. (1964), *A Short History of Midwifery*, Philadelphia, PA:W. B. Saunders Company

Dewhurst, J (1980), *Royal Confinements*, London, UK:Weidenfeld and Nicolson

Eccles, A (1982), *Obstetrics and Gynaecology in Tudor and Stuart England*, London, UK:

Croom Helm Gelis, J (1991), *History of Childbirth: Fertility, Pregnancy and Birth in Early Modern Europe*, Boston, MA: Northeastern University Press

Green, MH. (2002), *The Trotula: A Medieval Compendium of Women's Medicine*, Philadelphia, PA: University of Pennsylvania Press

Musacchio, JM (1999), *The Art and Ritual of Childbirth in Renaissance Italy,* New Haven, CT: Yale University Press

Sharp, J (1999), *Midwives Book: Or the Whole Art of Midwifery Discovered*, New York, NY: Oxford University Press

www.ingramcontent.com/pod-product-compliance
Lightning Source LLC
Chambersburg PA
CBHW071158160426
43196CB00011B/2117